Find

ALTERNATIVE

M.D.s

Dr. Richard H. Leigh M.D.

Arle Hagberg

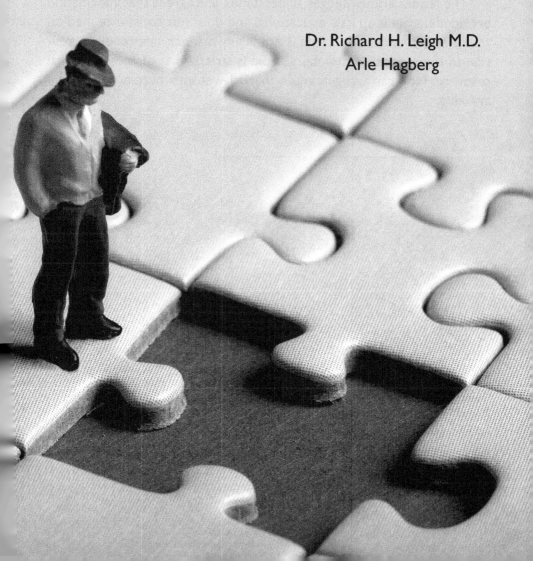

This manual of carefully selected research and e-sources was originally published as an e-book in 2003 by Wheelock Mountain Press of Vermont, Phillip Hurley, publisher.

Medical Disclaimer by the Authors:

The reader acknowledges, understands, and agrees that information provided herein is strictly educational and does not constitute medical advice in any manner. Dr. Leigh is not in any manner an attending physician to the reader. Ms. Hagberg's role is strictly that of an educational resource. Nor can we guarantee that all websites herein will remain available.

ISBN: 1451549709
ISBN-13: 9781451549706

Why another publication on Alternative Medicine? This directory is your "inside track" to state-of-the-art alternative medical resources, some of which are not available in other sources. For starters, the diagnostic skills of Emil Schandl, Ph.D., can accurately determine ten-twelve years in advance of the tumor www.CAprofile.net, but not leave you hanging in fear.

The web addresses provide instant access to key doctors, mostly in the United States, and other carefully selected web sites - an exponential base of information. Of course it was impossible to feature all of the talented medical resources and our apology to countless others whom you may locate from sources we list.

ƒThis resource will expedite your discovery of what truly may be your medical options. *However, bear in mind that it is not medical advice from either author.* Enjoy your exploration!

Acknowledgement... To the courageous medical pioneers of the 20th century who implemented non-surgical, drug-sparing methods in order to economize for their patients yet optimize their care. Currently over 3,000 U.S. physicians have embraced this legacy, now termed complementary or integrative medicine - the medical art of deciding when, and when not, to employ drugs and surgery.

The Authors

Richard H. Leigh, M.D., ACOG, ACAM, AAEM (ret), received his medical degree from the University of Illinois in 1948, interning at St. Luke's in Duluth, with residencies in obstetrics at St. Luke's, Fargo and University of Minnesota.

After medical service during the Korean Conflict, Dr. Leigh practiced Obstetrics and Gynecology in Grand Forks, North Dakota, until 1988. Guided by state of the art biochemical functional laboratory tests, Dr. Leigh then employed a comprehensive, antioxidant approach for mostly allergy and Chelation therapy patients until his retirement in 2006.

Arle Hagberg resides in Bemidji, Minnesota, and has researched medical doctors who use alternatives to drugs and surgery for 30 years. She assisted as a copy editor for James P. Carter, M.D., Dr. P.H., on his manuscript for _Racketeering in Medicine_, Hampton Roads Publishers, 1993.

Ms. Hagberg has education degrees in English, Social Studies, Sociology, and Learning Disabilities, and has a fascination for learning and teaching practical information from the consumer's viewpoint. The enclosed sources profess that medical costs could be reduced 50% by the full availability of the protocols in this sourcebook.

TABLE OF CONTENTS

Oral Chelation (tablets, sub-lingual, suppository)
3. American Academy for Environmental Medicine (AAEM)
4. International Society for Orthomolecular Medicine (ISOM)
   Nutrient approach to Psychiatric/Metabolic illness
5. International Gesellshaft für Cyto-Biologische Therapien e.V.
   (International Association for Live-Cell Therapy)
6. American Association of Orthopedic Medicine
7. American Rheumatoid Medical Association
8. International Oxidative Medical Association
   Hyperbaric Medical Association
   Bio-Immune, Inc.
9. American Association of Anti-Aging Medicine
10. Association for Comprehensive NeuroTherapy
11. The Cranial Academy
12. American College of Osteopathic Sclero-therapeutic
   Pain Management (ACOSPM)
13. Chiropractic Specialties:
   Gonstead, Cranial-Sacral, etc.
14. Homeopathic Medicine
15. College of Optometrists in Vision Development
16. American Academy of Medical Acupuncture
17. American Association of Naturopathic Physicians
18. Holistic Dental Association
19. Association of Natural Medicine Pharmacists
20. Foundation for the Advancement of Innovative Medicine
21. International College of Clinical Medicine
22. American Holistic Medical Association
23. American Holistic Nurses Association
24. Physician Association for Anthroposophical Medicine
25. International Tibetan Medical Association
26. International University for Alternative Medicines, Calcutta
27. Physicians for Photo Luminescence, Blood Irradiation
28. Physicians/Consultants for IPT (Insulin Potentiation Therapy)
29. Institute for Functional Medicine (IFM)
30. Altmeds for Alternative and Complementary Doctors
31. Breast Thermography:

Cognitive/Developmental Delay; Downs Syndrome;
Diabetes related;
Endometriosis; Eyes (Glaucoma, Macular, Cataract, etc.);
Fatigue;
Gender Needs and the Role of Nutrition and Hormonal Levels;
GERD (gastro-intestinal reflux disease); A Gastric Surgeon's alternative to his surgery; Gulf War Syndrome, Effects of Agent Orange on Vietnam Veterans;
Heart/Circulatory; Heavy Metals; Hepatitis; Huntington's Chorea;
IBS (Irritable Bowel Syndrome); Immune Therapy;
Indigestion; Infertility; Iron Overload;
Liver problems; Lupus; Lyme Disease;
Mental Health-Nutrition; Multiple Sclerosis;
Pain in Joints; Parkinson's; Post-Polio Syndrome; Prostate (BHP and Cancer of);
Structural - Bad Back, Limbs; SLE (Systemic Lupus Erythematosis);
Thyroid Conditions; Toxic Metal Syndrome;
Vaccination Side Effects; Vertigo (Dizziness, Imbalance); Vestibular-inner ear balance disorder; Vision (see eyes);
Yeast Syndrome: Men, Women, and Children;

Part 6 –
Appendices

Appendix 1. Insurance Coverage   77-78
-Alternative Health Insurance: alternative or conventional, your choice
-CareCredit® - No interest payment plans with participating doctors

Appendix 2. Dr. Leigh's Perspective on Supplements 79-80

Appendix 3. Reputable TV and Radio Resources 81-82

Part 1

Medicine Can't Afford Itself — Dr. Richard H. Leigh

We Need Complementary Medicine, as the current health care system in the United States can no longer afford itself. The prohibitive cost of conventional care affects our economy and American's health.

Complementary physicians estimate that full implementation of alternatives (when drugs and/or surgery are unnecessary) could reduce medical cost by fifty percent. In most cases, coronary by-pass at $50,000.00 can be replaced with I.V. Chelation for only a few thousand. This "workhorse" of alternative medicine alone could enable three-fourths of patients in nursing care to avoid this fate.

British Columbia psychiatrist and pioneer of Orthomolecular Medicine, Abram Hoffer, M. D., Ph.D., (deceased) asserted that he saved a province two million dollars for every schizophrenic patient treated with inexpensive nutrient therapy, a mild tranquilizer if needed, but only at the first office visit. Dr. Hoffer's breakthroughs in mental health treatment in the 1950's, stirred up a hornet's nest of criticism within the related conventional medical associations. www.doctoryourself.com, www.orthomolecular.org.

Proclamations that alternatives remain unproven through blinded studies are no excuse. It is common knowledge in medicine that 80-90% of medicine practiced had no blinded studies to justify efficacy

Several years ago, *The Townsend Letters for Doctors and Patients* www.townsendletter.com asserted that Health Science libraries receive over 4 million new pages per year from medical journals, most of which is excellent and relevant to clinical medicine:

"...No clinician (or even researcher) could possibly find the time to read one percent (40,000 pages/year) of the flood. Thus, we are all ignorant of the greatest findings. It might be stated that there is no area of human endeavor where ignorance (of what is known) is growing as rapidly as in clinical medicine. Hence, our ignorance is unavoidable but the arrogance and pretense of omniscience that we see so often in medicine today are philosophically inexcusable."

Alternative Medicine – more than herbs and acupuncture

In the hands of a skilled clinician, alternative treatments can heal or improve the patient, with no appreciable unwanted side effects, and often with longer lasting results. Case studies, valid empirical, clinical and research trials from all over the world attest to this.

World famous Oncology Surgeon, Francisco Contreras, clarified on Larry King, summer 2009, the validity for treating childhood Hodgkins with chemotherapy but in addition to the medical wisdom of "fractionated" chemotherapy (slow release over one-three days on I.V.) in conjunction with immune and nutritional support to achieve best results. This Onco-surgeon received five minute coverage a few times on a Saturday night in response to the recent media frenzy over a Minnesota mother fleeing with her child to "someplace" for natural treatment in Mexico, and repeated ad nauseum with no investigative reporting.

Alternative treatments often cost less than conventional treatments. Compare the cost of heart bypass surgery (can be $50,000+) to treating the same condition with a full series of IV chelation treatments ($2,000-$4,000). The chelation treatments often give more lasting results overall.

Unfortunately, Medicare is directed to finance costly, invasive procedures such as bypass and angioplasty but not to finance alternative treatments such as chelation. Recently, however, the states of Washington, West Virginia, Delaware and Maryland allow for Medicare coverage of Chelation.

The expensive, invasive procedures generally focus on the suppression of symptoms and have the potential for harmful side effects; whereas Chelation addresses the systemic nature of cardiovascular degeneration, gently removing the offending plaque and restoring circulation.

For more on Chelation, go to the first two entries in Part 3 - Medical Associations. A New York Chelation physician, Michael Schachter, has information on the "cheat-proof," NIH study pressured by chelation doctors, which was to conclude in 2008 www.mbschachter. Some years ago a blinded, controlled study by the VA on veterans was so favorable to chelation that the study was halted at mid-point in silence.

The paradigm shift towards a balanced use of drugs, surgery, and alternatives cannot be halted. However, the institutions in the United States that control health care remain fixated. U.S. health consumers should demand full availability of complementary (the combination of conventional and alternative) medicine.

Will the institutions that control the money accept alternatives in time? The know-how is already in place. Leaders in health insurance such as the California company, Alternative Health Insurance www.alternativeinsurance.com, and many other enterprising clinics and hospitals are already in operation.

Thousands of outpatient clinics in the United States already practice complementary medicine such as chelation. Standard lab work is used, sometimes with unique and more detailed interpretations. There is attention to detoxification on the cellular level, customized diets and key supplements with infusion therapy available for more effective results. This insurance company covers a subscriber's choice of conventional or alternative treatment for plaque buildup

Without national leadership to optimize the quality and reduce the cost of health care, consumers in a literate society must search on their own for medical professionals who can determine whether conventional or less expensive alternatives are preferable. The Foundation for the Advancement of Innovative Medicine, www.faim.org offers the reader a means to advance the civil right to choose.

Richard H. Leigh, M.D., ACOG, ACAM, AAEM (retired, 2006)

Grand Forks, ND

Part 2

Out of Europe: Stunning, Safe Medical Advances

Throughout the 20th century, drug-sparing and non-surgical, immune enhancing methods were developed in Europe, particularly Germany. These methods continue to be fine-tuned. Max Gerson was one of many German physicians involved in their development. Famous for his success in cancer therapy, he was praised by his friend, Dr. Albert Schweitzer, as a medical genius.

Gerson's approach was to dissolve malignancies by regenerating the body's own healing mechanisms. In *Gerson's Cancer Therapy: Results of Fifty Cases,* published in the 1950's (www.gerson.org), this medical pioneer foretold that prevention of chronic disease would be determined by family eating habits, agriculture practices, and methods of food preservation.

Today, Dr. Gerson would be pleased to observe the ongoing medical paradigm shift and the related commercial endeavors. For instance:

-Andrew Weil, M.D.'s demonstration of healthy cuisine to a nationwide audience on Oprah.

-Jordan Rubin, M.D.'s raw food chefs on his TBN programs www.jordanrubin.com as well as his tours throughout America with www.perfectweightamerica.com emblazoned on his gigantic bus.

-Nutrient formulas now being developed by all health care specialties, e.g., Dr. Gary Kappel, O.D.'s supplements for macular degeneration, glaucoma, cataracts, etc. Mrs. Kappel wrote a commendable guideline, *Food Preparation: Hints on Making it Happen* www.iquestsight.com.

-Former FDA attorney, Andrew Lessman's nutrition lessons on HSN, and certain ITV infomercials regarding nutritional supplements and, most recently, the integrative approach of NBC's Dr. OZ and Meet the Doctors.

However, Gerson arrived in mid 20th century when the power struggle was just heating up…

Dr. Gerson Comes to America
…But the public is shortchanged by four votes

Following a narrow escape from Nazi Germany, Dr. Gerson did not anticipate the rejection of his cancer protocol in the US. His success with American patients was astonishing, but the medical industry of that era was not interested.

In 1946, the doctor testified for three days before the Pepper-Neely Congressional Subcommittee. His testimony included extensive clinical proof, x-rays, lab results before/after of many of his cancer patients' full remissions. Conventional medicine had diagnosed these cases as "terminal," yet many of the patients lived for decades, some 40 years longer, following Gerson's treatments.

Despite the stunning medical success Dr. Gerson demonstrated, Senate Bill S.1875 (to determine the direction of government funding for cancer research) excluded funding for Gerson's approach. Intensive lobbying from special interests prevailed to obtain government funding for what is now conventional cancer treatments. Dr. Gerson's anticipation of a Nobel Prize in Medicine from his demonstration was never realized; instead he lost his cancer ward at Gotham Hospital, NY.

The Gerson Therapy survived, while another German legacy, the Issels Protocol (Dr. Joseph Issels) www.issels.com is available in a separate wing of the Oasis Hospital which is featured in this directory www.contrerashospital.com.

Medical Secrets - two of many

Alternative approaches depend on adequate immune function in the patient, in order to heal chronic degenerative diseases. Obviously, the earlier the alternative treatments begin, the more effective the results. Following are two relatively unknown treatments:

Prolotherapy – FDA-approved since 1947

Prolotherapy (nickname "prolo") repairs the connective tissue between joints. Also known as Reconstruction Injection Therapy (RIT), Prolotherapy (from proliferation of cells) is an established alternative to ankle, knee, hip, back, neck, and other joint surgery. This is an outpatient procedure that involves injecting nontoxic dextrose into a problem joint in order to stimulate (proliferate) the body's self-repair of connective tissue. The injections cause an inflammatory response stimulating collagen growth, which proliferates the re-growth and strengthens the ligaments and tendons, also cartilage.

Prolo alleviates pain and prevents surgery in the vast majority of cases. Endorsed and practiced at Virginia Tech, of the Atlantic Coast Conference, Prolo is catching on rapidly for healing sports and other injuries, including age related wear and tear. Prolo does not carry the political baggage of most alternatives and more orthopedic surgeons offer this treatment. We recommend for athletes, coaches, and parents to view Part 6 - Appendix 4 on Prolo.

European Live Cell Therapy – for those who happen to discover it

Modern use of this endocrine approach began in the 1930's when Swiss physician Paul Niehans expanded on the earlier research of Kuttner (circa 1912). By accident, a colleague of Niehans excised (cut out) the parathyroid of a woman whose condition then deteriorated to near death as she waited for a transplant. Niehans injected her with a suspension of tissue cells (a splice of) from a young ox. This injection restored her condition, and the patient lived for another 24 years.

Convinced, Niehans developed corresponding fetal glandular cells and organ extracts from cattle and sheep, which were eventually raised for that purpose. Intramuscular injections of these extracts stimulated significant cognitive development (Franz Schmid) and physical development in congenital, heritable conditions, and in numerous chronic and acute problems. See Part 3 - Medical Association #5.

7

Niehans later shifted his focus to anti-aging restoration for the rich and famous, but his landmark contributions for recoveries in congenital, neurological, chronic, and acute conditions are well documented; and the treatments he developed are still in use today. Unfortunately, his breakthroughs were sensationalized by the press, which even back then didn't do their homework and he failed to utilize patenting procedures to claim credit for his discovery.

Research and clinical use of live-cell therapy continued, eventually with preserved cell tissue (as opposed to fresh) but never human cells. The preserved forms varied in efficacy. Unscrupulous doctors developed Inferior medical imitations that were marketed by business interests. This problem continues today, so buyer beware.

Dr. Niehans' *Introduction to Cellular Therapy* was first published in English, in 1960. A summary of his works and the work of others in the field, entitled *Cell Research and Cellular Therapy* was published in English in 1967.

Live Cell treatment for developmentally delayed children
Dr. Franz Schmid (deceased) directed the Kinderklinik in Aschaffenburg, Germany, and pursued research in live cell treatment for the developmentally delayed, claiming significant increase in I.Q. and other physical normalization. Case studies can be found in Schmid's *Das Mongolismus-Syndrom.*

The doctors practicing this treatment do not guarantee cognitive and physical development, but improvement usually occurs. In older children, cognitive development is generally 20-30 I.Q. points. Injections can begin as early as 8 lbs. and 8 weeks old. It was observed by an Ontario parent, while in Germany, that treatment at two months can result in obvious facial normalizing within several days.

Generally, the younger the child, the more effective is the treatment. The injections may be administered up to adolescence with improvements and minimal, if any, side effects, but the treatment is most effective in the first decade of life.

Americans access Live Cell Therapy in Germany

Live cell therapy is an established medical specialty in Germany. There are two U.S. contacts in this directory for Americans interested in pursuing such treatment abroad. One is a liaison between inquiring parents and the members of a German Medical Association, Internationale Gesellschaft für Cyto-biologische Therapien eV. (International Association for Cellular Research) located in Waldorf, Germany. See Part 3 - Medical Association #5.

The other U.S. contact is a parent support group. Some members of this group who could afford travel to Germany for the treatments, have arranged for families of more limited means to receive stateside consultation from a German doctor.

Until his death, Dr. Schmid generously treated American children with developmental delay at no charge, professing his gratitude for the role of the U.S. military in Germany during World War II. In the doctor's words, "...For saving us from ourselves."

Schmid, Niehans and other esteemed European medical pioneers were discouraged from presenting their studies and findings to the U.S. medical establishment, and thus from sharing their success with American health care consumers.

For instance, the nontoxic Calcium Orotate formula of famous German doctor, Hans Nieper, was not approved in the U.S. despite its value in treating multiple sclerosis without side-effects.

www.naturalhealthconsult.com/Monographs/calEAP.html

Dr. Wolfram W. Kühnau

A disciple of Niehans, Dr. Kühnau, (deceased) immigrated to the U.S. in the 1980's and offered cellular injection treatment at the respected American Biologics Hospital in Mexico, (no longer in operation). Taking advantage of the local resources Dr. Kühnau would gather the embryonic sacks of Blue Sharks caught by coastal fishermen. He found first trimester blue shark embryo to be a superior cellular source, and he incorporated this in his treatment. Dr. Velasques of Mexico, has a similar practice.   www.extendlife.com

First trimester embryo tissue is not yet imprinted with an immune system for a host reaction, nor is it site and organ specific. Unencumbered by the health and moral issues of human stem cell usage, Dr. Kühnau contributed to Niehans' *Die Zellulartherapie* in 1954. Dr. Kühnau's readable monograph about cellular therapy, <u>*Live Cell Therapy (Xenotransplants): My life with a Medical Breakthrough,*</u> is currently out of print but used copies may be available on www. Amazon.com.

Dr. Kühnau was involved with the International Spinal Cord Regeneration Center (ISRC), collaborating with Neurosurgeon Carlos Romero Gaitan and Orthopedic Surgeon Fernando Ramirez del Rio in ongoing research in a promising spinal cord rejuvenation program. To date, their success is only with spinal cord injuries that are referred to as 'complete,' meaning absence of any sensory and motor function below the site injury. SEVERED SPINAL CORD CASES ARE NOT ACCEPTED at this time. Candidates are conservatively screened so that their current level of health is not jeopardized. Not all of the screened patients respond, but there have been sufficient recoveries for the treatment to be considered a viable medical option.

The ISCR website http://spinal.siteutopia.net   is informative and thorough, and offers a DVD on spinal cord rejuvenation. It includes a Patient Recovery Data Section, chart indicating the Postulated Modes of Action, and a FAQ with clear, honest and detailed answers. There is also a profound discussion of the reluctance of the U.S. medical establishment
to approve or even consider medical treatments that are accepted and available in Europe and Mexico.

One of the ISCR patients who received embryonic cell transplant therapy had a website under construction:

http://mzonpy e.mweb.co.za/residents/dhouston/indes.html

The treatment for paralysis consists of a multi-faceted, complementary approach which combines conventional neurosurgery and orthopedic surgery, with injections of drugless animal embryonic cells:

-Traditional decompression surgery to reconstruct the spinal canal.

-Microsurgery to remove typical scarring, cysts, fragments.

-Insertion of a permanent shunt for draining cysts.

-Injections of live embryonic cells that will gradually re-grow the neural matrix across the injury site.

-Subsequent cell treatments at progressively lower levels of the cord to reverse cord atrophy from lack of use or reduced nutritional ingredients carried by activated spinal fluid.

-Application of scarring inhibitors and growth enhancing factors including remyelination.

-Patient cooperation is essential in physical therapy and nutrition components.

In the current clamor for stem cell research funding, little is said about the high stakes interest in patent profits and royalties. In the mainstream, primary research goals involve reproduction, cloning, etc., but proponents also point toward goals in the treatment of genetic, congenital, neurological, and chronic maladies to further justify their mega-funding requests.

Both the immune-enhancing methods of Gerson, et al; and Niehans' animal embryo cellular injections demonstrate great promise in the areas mentioned above. Still, the U.S. medical establishment largely ignored cost-effective, drugless immune therapy, and live cell injections from non-human sources.

Stem cell proponents in the U.S. seem oblivious to the warnings of cellular experts who oppose the use of non-host human tissue to treat humans at any life stage.

Dr. Kuhnau on the medical risks of using human tissue

In his readable and fascinating book; *Live CellTherapy (Xenotransplants): My Life with a Medical Breakthrough*, Dr. Kühnau explains the potential medical risks of using human tissue to treat human patients.

Quote, courtesy of Dr. Wolfram Kühnau, offered during our phone conversation a few years before his passing:

"The American press has devoted a great deal of time and space to a discussion of the use of embryonic human tissue from legal abortions and the creation of a so-called "tissue bank" for treatment of humans with this tissue.

I have no desire to discuss any moral considerations of this proposal. I do, however, wish to discuss the scientific and medical ramifications.

There are four compelling reasons why human tissue should never be used to treat humans:

1. It is impossible to be 100% certain that the human tissue which might be used would be free of either the HIV virus and/or the mutant strains of the AIDS virus which now are surfacing. It is now well known that the test for AIDS can read absolutely negative and a later test can show positive.

2. The comments in No.1 apply as well to the test for the Hepatitis B Virus.

3. The same comments are appropriate to the test for Hepatitis C Virus.

4. With the use of human tissue there is always the possibility of producing a 'Kuru', a hopelessly deadly disease which is still found in

remote areas such as Papua, New Guinea where ritual cannibalism is still practiced.

Dr. Gaydusek received the Nobel Prize in Medicine for describing this disease. Initially it was believed that a virus alone was the cause of Kuru*. Now we know that auto-immunological factors can play a major role in these tragic cases. Since we humans have receptors for human material and animals do not, and because all of the above four mentioned negatives do not exist, e.g., in the shark, it is simply logical that animal tissue is far superior to human tissue and should be the material of choice.

To repeat, animal (fetal) tissue taken in the early stages of pregnancy is very well tolerated and when used in a reasonable and conscientious manner is usually risk free. Pregnant cows beyond number are slaughtered daily and sharks are hunted and killed daily. In both cases the embryonic sac is normally thrown away as worthless. The shortsightedness of the medical community in this regard is particularly tragic in their refusal to consider these highly effective materials.

Now you may ask about the possibility of transmitting animal diseases to humans with these implants. The easiest way to avoid this possibility is to very carefully control the material being used. In Mexico undulant fever and other cattle diseases do not exist. Beef leukemia does not exist here.

Live cell therapy opens a new door in medicine; one that does not permit the fallacious excuse that in the "incurable case" nothing can be done. A superb example of this is evidenced by the fact that the two Germans who were the latest Nobel Prize winners in medicine had discovered that on the surface of the cell there are channels of such a fine dimension that they will allow only ions (electrically active particles) to pass to the next cell.

So in the official "Laudatio" of the Nobel Prize Committee, it was pointed out that Drs. Sakman and Neher are working on new "drugs" which are enabling us to fight effectively against genetic diseases. As an example, cystic fibrosis was mentioned."

End of quote, Dr. Kühnau

FOOTNOTE: *Kuru is the native term for CJD (Creutzfeldt Jakob Disease), an agonizing, neurological disintegration resulting from consumption of same species in any form. It is not always discernible in the lab and capable of "hiding" within the cell.

The Western form of Kuru: CJD

In Germany, the same problem arose, also conditioned by cultural factors, but involving the hallmarks of an advanced industrial culture: medicine, manufacturing and marketing.

In the winter of 2002, a documentary on CBC Canada, www.cbc.ca exposed a scandal involving the illegal acquisition, processing, and distribution of a cadaver-derived, dural tissue material by which to patch certain surgical incisions in the brain.

The raw dura (protective tissue surrounding the brain) was illegally harvested from cadavers, without informing loved ones or filing requests for tissue donation. A German pharmaceutical company manufactured the patch material by mass pooling the cadaver tissues with no regard for proper sterilization. The manufactured product was then distributed worldwide, retailing for $340.00 per square inch patch. Unsuspecting surgeons appreciated the convenience of this natural, surgical patch, commercial name Lyodura, in place of the usual skin grafts from the involved patient.

Following an "incubation period" of a decade, certain brain surgeries from 1972 - 1989, were eventually and quietly tied to subsequent outbreaks of the devastating and always terminal CJD (Creutzfeldt Jakob Disease).

Throughout the CBC interview, the Montreal based distributor remained adamant as to his lack of culpability in its distribution. Fortunately, this convenient surgical bandage never made it through the rigors of FDA approval and was applied only minimally in the

Northeastern United States before the FDA fulfilled its intended role of protecting the American public.

Alternative Medicine - Available in Europe and Mexico, less in the US

Worldwide throughout the 20th Century, affluent health consumers sought alternative care in Europe. Many of these European alternative medical centers were spa related. Highly regarded and staffed with qualified health care professionals, they continue to attract patients of means.

In the past 30 years, clustered in the Northern Baja (the Tijuana area of Mexico near the U.S. border), there has been steady growth of health care centers patterned after those of Europe. This medical concentration has come about for a number of reasons:

The nontoxic treatments for reversal of chronic, degenerative diseases are not "approved" in the United States without a 4 to 8 hundred million dollar blinded study for each protocol. Ironically, 80-90% of conventional American medical procedures lack that exorbitant form of proof. The policy of the Mexican government allows unconventional therapies that have no demonstrated harmful side effects.

The border proximity to U.S. patients, most of whom cannot afford the higher costs of travel to Europe for alternative treatment. Northwestern Mexico (Tijuana area) has convenient access from all points in the U.S., and from the rest of the world, via LA International. Patients are met by their designated medical van at the baggage counters at the airport and returned after their treatment time, ranging from several days to several weeks. However, the eminent Contreras Hospital now serves patients in Irvine, California.

The economy of Mexico provides much lower cost for quality health care at the centers. A spouse or loved one may have room and board at no or very low cost with the patient in hospital, and excellent, nutritious food is also available.

Many patients do not require hospitalization, so on both sides of the border, honest business owners of small motels, camping and R.V. sites accommodate the continuous flow of outpatients who choose to return to the United States after morning treatments. Often, motel owners provide facilities and services that assist the patient in daily routines of special diet and detoxification.

The medical facilities range from full hospitals to small outpatient clinics. Licensed, highly experienced doctors out of Europe, the United States, Mexico, other Latin American countries, and Asia, staff quality health care centers that use European-based alternatives to drugs/surgery for all manner of chronic, degenerative diseases. Doctors, nurses, and administrators often commute from their homes located in the San Diego area.

The treatment centers usually have offices in the United States for patient inquiry, and they advertise in some alternative health publications, such as www.alternativemedicine.com.

Their demonstrated success in reversing even "terminal" conditions (those given up on in conventional cancer centers in Europe and the United States) is impressive; especially when one considers that many of their patients are advanced and have compromised immune systems from the effects of chemotherapy and radiation and the progression of the disease itself.

For those whose terminal condition cannot be arrested, quality of life without pain is competently addressed with nontoxic pain relief. It must be emphasized that alternative medicine depends on a sufficiently functioning immune system in order to work, so the earlier in the disease cycle that alternative treatments begin, the more effective they are.

Should Americans have to leave their own country for effective, inexpensive, and nontoxic treatments that have demonstrated efficacy, safety and modest cost? Are doctors in other countries innately more capable than ours? Should the drug and criminal elements associated with Mexico automatically negate the value of these internationally respected hospitals and clinics? Certainly not, **but with the recent drug related border violence, inquiries should be made before crossing.**

Buyer beware

Occasionally, con artists try to impersonate doctors that belong to the thriving medical alternative (and conventional) community in Tijuana. To avoid such enterprising criminals, some of whom are U.S. citizens, the authors have listed in Part 4 – Prominent Treatment Centers, several of the most prestigious of the thirty alternative medical centers in the Tijuana area that have established reputations.

The venerable non-profit www.cancercontrolsociety.com of Los Angeles, lists these medical centers and sponsors an annual Labor Day convention of alternative doctors, recovered cancer patients, and lay people. This includes a doctors' symposium for the public. Satisfied patients in our sources can help the consumer learn of the wide range of reputable choices, both within and beyond the United States. See Part 4 – Prominent Treatment Centers.

Insurance may pay 80% of the treatment costs, but may be allowed to do so only in hospital settings. Alternative Insurance (www.alternative insurance.com) is one progressive insurance company that allows freedom of choice. Payment is required on arrival, but the attending hospital can recommend an agency to process your insurance claim for timely reimbursement.

Real quackery or just propaganda?

U.S. physicians, who employ drug/surgery sparing methods within their scope of practice, have faced prolonged disciplinary actions despite their documented success. Health consumers may encounter generalized libelous statements in print or slanderous remarks regarding these medical facilities, but rarely are they mentioned by name. Such untruths are propagated in the media by those who have never accepted the standing offers of the alternative medical establishments in question to investigate their medical files.

To add to the confusion, sound-bite presentations in the media infer that alternative medicine is simply 'herbs, acupuncture, massage, visualization, or having a nice day with no acknowledgement that alternative treatments may combine conventional treatments performed by licensed medical staff with membership in reputable medical associations. Consumers must separate the grain from chaff by their own careful investigation.

Sinister imitators, a chilling example

In the winter of 2002, a CBC (Canadian Broadcasting Company) documentary featured the story of an immigrant couple from Eastern Europe who sought alternative cancer care. Upon her diagnosis of breast cancer, they were misled by a health food center in the province of Manitoba, Canada that connected them with a 'cancer clinic' in Mexico, where they were preyed upon.

They arrived in Mexico to an empty house that lacked a posted address and she was administered some sort of ozone like therapy that initially made her feel improvement. Whether contraband or contrived, ozone alone cannot heal without a total medical plan. Her condition quickly worsened over a few weeks. Supposedly, a "doctor" examined her upon her decline, but no one attended to her and there was no indication that this was a medical facility of any kind. Nor were there other patients in the facility.

The only indicated questioning on the part of this naive couple was their query for a house address. The next day one was posted to the entrance. They returned to Canada and she soon expired.

CBC documentaries enjoy a tradition for in-depth analysis and perspectives from both sides of an issue. Where was their usual approach to an issue that would have exposed how this quackery originated from a deadly imitation of the reputable medical community? There are many satisfied Canadian patients willing to attest to their personal satisfactory treatments at reputable medical establishments in Mexico. Or, a spokes-person from one of the reputable medical centers could have been interviewed to expose the fact that con artists ply on their good name.

Unfortunately, the media fears commercial and licensing backlash from the powers that be. Otherwise, there would be solid documentary coverage of what flourishes south of the border and it would eliminate this aspect of medical fraud.

Medical turf wars that resort to libel and slander of alternative approaches in Western medicine have always waged. Even in Germany, where alternatives originated, doctors actually mass produced pamphlets to libel none other than Dr. Hans Nieper for his nontoxic, effective treatment for multiple sclerosis!

With the recent death of Dr. Nieper, his medical legacy will hopefully continue in Dr. Joachim Ledwoch's practice www.dr-ledwoch. de and Dr. med. Peter Wolf www.hyperthermia-center-hannover. com. Dr. Nieper's legacy and those who adhere to it are thoroughly documented in the Brewer Archive, Richland, Wisconsin www.mwt. net/~drbrewer.

It is doubtful that Dr. Nieper's colleagues will be any more welcome in the United States, but if a health consumer with M.S. learns of this alternative in time (within four years of diagnosis) and can afford to cross the Atlantic, he/she may still be treated by the safe, effective Nieper protocol.

Currently other U.S. doctors are effectively managing, even reversing chronic illnesses. For more info, go to Drs. Perlmutter and Hoffman at www.perlmutter.com or www.drhoffman.com.

Dr. Nieper also had impressive success in treating cancer and heart disease patients from all over the world with natural therapies. One therapy developed by Dr. Nieper was the daily ingestion of silkworm derived tablets to dissolve arterial plaque. Chelation doctors themselves should note this potential alternative or adjuvant to infusion Chelation for dissolving plaque.

An American medical center denies the existence of a former patient

A final irony involved a paralysis patient. Initially seen by a conventional paralysis treatment center in the U.S. with no benefit, the patient achieved significant improvement at the International Spinal Cord

Regeneration Center http://spinal.siteutopia.net. Upon his return to the US center, his past existence as a patient there was denied, according to the assertion at this website:

A federally funded US research facility on paralysis...

"...when presented with a patient of ours who had demonstrated new levels of functional ability (the facility in question) denied that it had occurred...

...even though the patient was originally diagnosed at that facility as being 'complete' (paralyzed from point of injury down to end of spine) and the progress is documented by both EMG results and by a renewed lifestyle."

Part 3 – Medical Associations

1. American College for Advancement in Medicine (ACAM)
Laguna Hills, California www.acam.org

ACAM is one of two medical associations that determine protocol for the administration of I.V. Chelation. ACAM provides physician locations by state; also books and media to purchase.

FDA approved in 1947, U.S. medical doctors have used I.V. Chelation Therapy to remove heavy metal accumulation in the circulatory system. Over 1,000 ACAM members practice in the U.S. while over 500 practice in other countries, mostly Canada, Europe, and the America's. 1-800-532-3688 if unable to locate at website.

The original use resulted in this discovery: what removed heavy metal toxins also removed arterial plaque. Eventually, this viable alternative to by-pass surgery, angioplasty, and various heart/circulatory meds, will be routine medical practice.

Many chelation doctors have informative websites, their own books, and media for other conditions as well. The NIH (National Institute of Health) was pressured into a cheat-proof eight year study which was to end in 2008. Dr. Schachter offers further information on this study at www.mbschachter.com and "The next page features the second medical association for Chelation Therapy, ABCMT."

Find **ALTERNATIVE** M.D.s

Not all competent chelation doctors belong to ACAM. For example, in Minnesota, west of St. Cloud in Sartell, Dr. Thomas Sult practices chelation and a variety of complementary care www.icareclinics.com.

Drs. Leigh and Cranton and other sources will further define the "work horse" of alternative medicine.

2. The American Board of Clinical Metal Toxicology

Chicago, Illinois www.abcmt.org

This board determines the qualifications for certification in the field of Clinical Metal Toxicology. The website provides an interesting history and present day perspective on the role of heavy metals in promoting diseases.

The International Board of Clinical Metal Toxicology is headquartered in The Netherlands www.ibcmt.org

Both websites provide fascinating histories and information on the relationship of heavy metals to chronic health. The proper removal of mercury-based dental fillings (biological dentistry) and the careful removal of mercury and other heavy metals from the arteries (chelation) are two good examples of related alternative approaches.

Age Management Medicine Group www.agemed.org

(Hormone optimization is one approach)

The Institute of Functional Medicine www.functionalmedicine.org

(Personalized medicine that deals with primary prevention and underlying causes, instead of symptoms for chronic diseases)

International Academy of Oral Medicine and Toxicology www.iaomt.org

(Science-based biological dentistry)

Dr. Leigh defines I.V. Chelation:

"Chelation Therapy is a treatment program designed to improve blood flow through the arteries. It includes an infusion of EDTA, a chemical commonly used in the food industry as an emulsifier. Ethylene-diamine-tetra-acetic acid is a synthetic amino acid). It was

23

developed by the Germans after World War II to treat poison gas injury. In the early 1950's, EDTA was found effective in clearing heavy metals, such as mercury cadmium, and lead, from the body.

Quite by accident while performing this therapy, attending doctors made a significant observation: the ulcerated sores on patients' legs also healed! This discovery led to the concept of utilizing a chemical means to treat the damages caused by arterial atherosclerosis.

Atherosclerosis is a disease acquired over a period of years. It is an ongoing accumulation of fatty plaques in the arteries. When these plaques reach a certain thickness, a reduction in blood flow results, causing decreased circulation, pain and loss of strength. This can be incapacitating and even life threatening. This is a problem that will usually be with you for the rest of your life.

This treatment, (like that for diabetes mellitus) will be variably successful, depending upon several factors: your genetic inheritance; pretreatment level of illness; and your willingness to change your eating habits and lifestyle.

The symptoms of atherosclerosis are many but the most visible are:

- Those related to angina, which is coronary artery pain.

- Claudication, which is the cramping that occurs in the calves when walking.

- Signs of skin ulceration and breakdown.
- Some have experienced association difficulties with vision (cataracts) and reduction in memory and mental acuity.

The treatment of I.V. Chelation usually involves up to 20 or more infusions, each lasting about three hours. This initial treatment program is recommended by ACAM, the medical organization dedicated to researching and promoting this approach to vascular health.

It has been shown that after any treatment is concluded, there will be continued improvement for about three months. Generally, follow-up

treatments are governed by the patients' own symptoms. It is my recommendation that follow-up treatments be considered as soon as there is a decline in energy or increase in pain. Usually, one or two treatments per month suffice to maintain one's level of comfort.

My own clinic followed the carefully designed protocol set by ACAM. The traditionally safe, 3 grams of EDTA with each infusion is used. In addition, we use numerous vitamins and other helpful additives that are designed to meet individual needs.

(There are two forms of EDTA: the original Magnesium EDTA which takes 3 hours for infusion and Calcium EDTA, the latest form used by Dr. Leigh prior to retirement and takes only about one hour).

Nutrition is of major importance. Minerals, vitamins, digestive enzymes, and stomach hydrochloric acid are especially necessary in the older individual for proper digestion and utilization of foods eaten. Without these nutrients present in the proper amounts, maximum benefit from chelation is not possible. To reiterate, these are recommended on an individual basis.

The use of I.V. chelation throughout the second half of the 20th century has been politically controversial, despite the obvious benefit and outstanding safety record. As with any medical procedure, I.V. chelation must be performed by a physician trained in the rigorous protocol that is espoused by ACAM, the original medical association with expertise in this strictly medical procedure or by ABCMT."

Dr. Cranton's website www.drcranton.com is an in-depth resource for Chelation and other chronic, degenerative conditions. From the doctor's website:

"Intravenous chelation therapy with ethylene diamine tetra-acetic acid (EDTA) is proven to reverse and slow the progression of atherosclerosis and age-related diseases. Symptoms affecting many different parts of the body often

Atherosclerotic blockage to blood flow in the coronary arteries of the heart, to the brain, to the legs, and elsewhere are relieved.

Blood flow increases. Heart attacks, strokes, leg pain and gangrene are prevented using this therapy. Bypass surgery and balloon angioplasty can often be prevented.

Under a carefully monitored program of a certified chelation physician, it is possible to avoid bypass surgery and amputation from gangrene; normalize cholesterol, triglycerides, and many other symptoms of cardio-vascular disease. Published studies now indicate that even cancer deaths can

be reduced by EDTA chelation
therapy."

Dr. Cranton answers questions in-depth for professional and laypersons. Note his latest edition of _Bypassing Bypass Surgery._ His clinics are located in Troutdale, WVA, and Yelm, WA. Alzheimer's and related conditions have been treated as well.

What about Oral Chelation?
(tablet by mouth, or sublingual under the tongue)

There is some disagreement among certain chelation specialists regarding this newer approach. We mention this topic out of concern for the growing number of oral Chelation formulas that are advertised with no apparent connection to a Chelation physician.

One exception is Dr. Garry Gordon, Payson, Arizona (Gordon Research Institute: www.gordonresearch.com) who is a practicing I.V. Chelation physician and has an oral chelation formula (www.longevityplus.net). If one is contemplating oral chelation, it would be advisable to seek out a physician of his expertise. Dr. Gordon is also featured on TV infomercials for Iceland Health and Omega 3 fish oil products www.icelandhealth.com, for conditions other than cardio-vascular. Dr. Gordon is quoted on the front cover of this directory.

Another reliable source for an oral formula, is British physician Thomas Smith who has worked with Dr. Nieper's silkworm enzyme derivative, serratia peptidase, in oral form for dissolving plaque.

www.icbr.com/reg2.htm

The authors recommend direct involvement by an appropriate health care physician. At the end of his career, Dr. Leigh was also investigating a sub-lingual form of oral chelation to avoid the interference from passing through the digestive system. Other means such as anal suppositories are available for chelation, and this is now endorsed by the prominent naturopath, Valerie Saxion, N.D. who appears weekly on TBN's "Alternative Health." www.valeriesaxion.com

Do you know your Homo-Cysteine level? Your C-RP level?

Dallas physician, Dr. Kenneth Cooper, M.D., M.P.H., discussed the importance of the indicators Homo-Cysteine and C-RP on his "Healthy Living" weekly radio show. Dr. Cooper also emphasizes exercise and aerobics for cardiovascular fitness. www.cooperwellness.com

Homo-Cysteine is an amino acid that assists dairy and animal protein assimilation. The C-Reactive Protein level measures systemic irritation or infection, which is a coronary risk factor. According to Dr. Cooper:

Homo-Cysteine levels:	9 or less is desirable.
10-13	normal but ascending risk for heart attack.
14	considered an unsafe level.

The C-Reactive Protein level: A C-RP level of .6-1 is a desirable range, the lower the better.

Homo-Cysteine: Important New Risk Factor in Cardiovascular Disease

By John Reynolds, PA-C, CCN www.mbschachter.com link on Homo-Cysteine)

Multivitamins as effective agents to lower homocysteine levels: www.heart-health.org/ArchIntMed3-2001.htm

Dr. Walker's first book on chelation, Everything You Should Know about Chelation, relates the fascinating account of how three doctors, Drs. Frankel, Tavel, and Hohnbaum, saved their lives with this intravenous procedure.

Dr. Hohnbaum, scheduled for next day, double-foot amputation, saved both his feet from amputation. View his dramatic before/after pictures of diabetic feet recovery that improved within days of his first treatment in October, with full recovery between November and February.

View the illustrated chapter provided on the above doctor-patients at Amazon and purchase there or from the publisher. This highly respected medical writer encountered powerful opposition upon its publication in the early 1980's. www.amazon. com www.drmortonwalker.com.

"Politics of Chelation" discussion with Gary Null, Ph.D. and an RN/BSN

www.garynull.com/Documents/Chelation_Therapy. htm

Dr. James R. Privatera has a clinic in California and has published the books:

Heart Attack: How to Prevent One and

Silent Clots: Life's Biggest Killer www.nutriscreen.com

Dr. Steenblock provides ozone treatments for stroke, traumatic brain injury, cerebral palsy, and other neurological conditions

www.strokedoctor.com

Dr. Michael Schachter's New York clinic www.mbschachter. com

Dr. Robert Cathcart's use of Vitamin C (ascorbic acid) in the treatment of many conditions   www.orthomed.com

Baxamed Clinics, Switzerland and New Delhi: www.baxamed. com

Drs. B.B. Singh and M. Mirchandani: Plaquex as an adjunct to I.V. Chelation: www.alternativehealthcenter.org

Dr. Dean Ornish has successfully used nutrition/life changes as an alternative even to I.V. Chelation Therapy! www.pmri.org

YOUR NOTES ON CHELATION:

3. American Academy of Environmental Medicine (AAEM)

Wichita, Kansas www.aaem.com

Members address treatments for environmental illness (E.I.), chemical sensitivity, hormone disruptors, allergies, and other reactions. What is environmental medicine, and environmentally triggered illnesses?

As defined by the AAEM website:

> "Environmental medicine is the comprehensive, proactive and preventive strategic approach to medical care dedicated to the evaluation, management, and prevention of the adverse consequences resulting from environmentally triggered illnesses.

> The model of environmental medicine is based on the growing appreciation that the human body is constantly coping with its dynamic environment by means of a number of inherited, built-in, complexly interacting, and usually reversible biological mechanisms and systems.

> Environmentally triggered illnesses (ETI) are the adverse consequences that result when the homodynamic interactions among biological functions are compromised by external or internal stressors. These stressors may range from severe acute exposure to a single stres-

sor, to cumulative relatively low-grade exposures to many stressors over time.

The resultant dysfunction is dependent on the patient's genetic make-up, his nutrition and health in general, the stressors, the degree of exposure to them and the effects of seven fundamental biological governing principles, biochemical individuality, individual susceptibility, the total load, the level of adaptation, the bipolarity of responses, the spreading phenomenon, and the switch phenomenon."

Note: Environmental illness physicians use serum antibody testing to detect present and previous toxic accumulation that embeds permanently in the lymphocytes.

Following are Important sources on Environmental Illness, endocrine (hormone) disruption:

Environmental Health Center Dallas www.ehcd.com

Environmental Working Group www.ewg.org

American Environmental Health Foundation www.aehf.com

Multiple Chemical Sensitivity and Chemical Injury http://bcn.boulder.co.us/health/rmeha/rmersrc.htm

Dr. Sherry Rogers' books; and mold detection kits www.prestigepublishing.com

Not Under My Roof is a video for protecting babies from toxins at home. Center for Children's Health and the Environment www.childenvironment.org

More sources on the issue of endocrine (hormone) disruption:

Raising Healthy Children in a Toxic World www.ourstolenfuture.org

Children's Environmental Health Network
www.cehn.org
Mercury Detoxification   www.healing-arts.org/children/
amyholmes.htm 58 pages, get rid of pests w/out chemicals
www.beyondpesticides.org
www.seventhgen.com

Research Foundation of Broda Barnes, M.D.
www.brodabarnes.org

DAMS, Intl. (Dental Amalgam Mercury Solutions)
1043 Grand Avenue #317
St. Paul, MN 55105
1-651-633-4572   or dams@usfamily.net

On request, DAMS has available scientific and educational publications on dental amalgam filling and related subjects; resources by state or province.

See also entry #18 - Holistic Dental Association;
www.mercurypoisoned.com and www.toxicteeth.com

Is there a threat created by drug-contaminated water?

According to an article by Greg Schilhab, editor, Quarterly Newsletter of the Canadian Schizophrenia Foundation, Winter 2001:

"Anti-biotics, anti-depressants, birth control pills, seizure medication, cancer treatments, pain killers, tranquilizers and cholesterol-lowering compounds have all been detected in Ontario water sources. The 30-60 most commonly prescribed pharmaceuticals are now attracting attention as a potentially new class of environmental contamination."

4. International Society for Orthomolecular Medicine (ISOM)

Toronto, Ontario

Members are in the practice of Orthomolecular Medicine or Orthomolecular Psychiatry. Many of the doctors maintain clinic websites. www.orthomed.org provides an interesting perspective entitled,

"Principles that Identify Orthomolecular Medicine" by Ortho. Psy., Richard Kunin, San Francisco. ISOM defines orthomolecular medicine as:

> "...the practice of preventing and treating disease by providing the body with optimal amounts of substances which are natural to the body. The term 'orthomolecular' (proper molecules) was first used by Linus Pauling in a paper he wrote in the journal, Science, in 1968. This paper first described the theoretical foundations for what was later to become a specialty within complementary medicine.
>
> The key idea in orthomolecular medicine is that genetic factors are central not only to the physical characteristics of individuals, but also to their biochemical milieu. Biochemical pathways of the body have significant variability in terms of transcriptional potential and individual enzyme concentrations, receptor-ligand affinities and protein transporter efficiency.

Diseases such as atherosclerosis, cancer, schizophrenia or depression are associated with specific biochemical abnormalities that are either causal or aggravating factors of the illness.

In the orthomolecular view, it is possible that the provision of vitamins, amino acids, trace elements or fatty acids in amounts sufficient to correct biochemical abnormalities will be therapeutic in preventing or treating such diseases."

Canadian Schizophrenia Foundation

16 Florence Avenue, Toronto, ON M2N 1E9
Tel 416-733-2117/Fax 416-733-2352 www.orthomed.org

The Canadian Schizophrenic foundation (CSF) produced *Masks of Madness: Science of Healing* ($39.95 includes GST/s/h). This 50 minute documentary features Psychiatrist Abram Hoffer, also Drs. Patrick Holford, Hugh Riordan, Hyla Cass, Gradford Weeks, Michael Janson, et.al.

In this documentary, the doctors recount their therapeutic approach, their satisfaction at seeing patients recover from the "incurable," as well as the professional resistance they faced when incorporating orthomolecular medicine into their medical and psychiatric practices.

Former patients (including Lois Lane actress, Margot Kidder, as host) participate in a candid roundtable discussion of their individual descents into mental illness; their difficulties in getting answers from conventional psychiatry; and their final recoveries using diet, supplements, and minimal pharmacological intervention.

The following publication topics can be purchased from CSF (usually under $5.00):

* Alcohol and drug abuse
* Allergies, sensitivities and ecologic illness
* Biosocial studies (juvenile behaviors influenced by allergy and diet)
* Candida albicans
* Cancer
* Immune system issues
* Cardiovascular conditions
* Chelation treatment
* Food and diet
* Mental disorders including depression, Alzheimer's, stress, and schizophrenia
* Trace elements, mineral analysis, and vitamin and mineral supplementation.
* General and orthomolecular topics

Orthomolecular Medicine Journal

Editor-in-Chief, Dr. Abram Hoffer, M.D., Ph.D., (deceased) The 'Godfather' of Orthomolecular Psychiatry, an esteemed medical pioneer. $55.00 US annual. Dr. Hoffer's quotes appear on the front cover of this directory. www.orthomed.org

Dr. Hoffer's publications can be reviewed and purchased at www.doctoryourself.com. A term search for abram hoffer, books, nutrition will uncover countless interviews, articles, books about his success in reversing depression, schizophrenia, bi-polar, etc., when patients cooperate with easy-to-follow supplement and diet protocols. Dr. Hoffer may have prescribed only a mild tranquilizer at the initial visit for schizophrenic patients under duress; control over schizophrenia is usually achieved within a few days. Dr. Hoffer's Curriculum Vitae:
www.healthy.net/bios.hoffer/CV.htm
Hoffer's Home page, "Orthomolecular Treatment of Cancer"
www.islandnet.com

Pfeiffer Treatment Center of Illinois, Minnesota www.hripct.org

Effects of biochemistry on behavior, thought and mood
Safe Harbor's resources, including doctors
www.alternativementalhealth.com

Dr. Cathcart's website www.orthmed.com
The Research Foundation of Dr. Broda Barne www.brodabarnes.org
Psychiatrist Daniel Amen on brain restoration through nutrition
www.amenclinics.com

5. Associations for European Live Cell Injection Therapies Xenotransplants (zen-o)

In Germany and Switzerland, animal embryo or fetal cells are harvested traditionally from lamb or calf (and recently blue shark embryo available in Mexico) then injected intra-muscular into the patient. This stimulates brain and physical development in genetic, congenital, chronic, and acute patients.

For fascinating descriptions and pictures before and after of children receiving these injections, buy Dr. Kühnau's book about live cell therapy. A video featuring surgeons assisting him in the treatment of spinal cord injuries.

http://spinal.siteutopia.net/

Dr. Kühnau's successor, Dr. Luiz Velazquez   www.extendlife.com

For I.Q. and other improvement in developmentally delayed children:

Internationale Gesellschaft für Cytobiologishche Therapien e.V.
(International Association for Cytobiological Therapies)
Dr. Fuchs, at Robert Bosch Strausse 56aD-69190 Waldorf, Germany

U.S. contacts for cell therapy can be located in Life Extension's directory of innovative clinics, Crystal Pines International Research Institute.
Dr. Fuch's listing follows in that directory.   www.lef.org
Other Sources for Live Cell Therapy:

Baxamed Clinics, Switzerland, New Delhi   www.baxamed.com

International Centers for Biological Recovery – Clinics that are licensed in the protocol of Dr. C. Thomas Smith, MD, HMD, D Hom (Med), PhD Nutritional Biochemistry. London, Nassau, Indonesia, and Mexico.
www.icbr.com

Arizona physician, Dr. Frank George's National Alliance Healthcare includes live cell. See also his international directory of organizations.
www.hbotofaz.org

Nevada Physician, Dr. Graham Simpson's Silent Inflammation Reduction
www.agelesszonereno.com

6. American Association of Orthopedic Medicine (AAOM)
Buena Vista, Colorado

Effective approaches to relieve acute and chronic pain emanating from the neck, mid-back, low-back, shoulder, elbow, wrist, hand, hip, knee, ankle, and feet.www.aaomed.org

This medical association educates physicians in the diagnosis and non-surgical treatment of musculo-skeletal problems. It promotes professional collaboration across multiple disciplines (integrative approach), including proliferate injections (Prolotherapy) which is defined at www.prolotherapy.com); steroid injections, fluoroscopic spinal interventions, osteopathic manual medicine, therapeutic exercise and interventions with various pharmaceuticals, nutraceuticals and hormones.

Find doctors by state who prevent joint surgery with Prolotherapy (non-toxic injections to stimulate healing) for stretched connective tissue for nearly all joint conditions for stretched ligaments, tendons, and cartilage. (See special appendix on sports injury.)
www.getprolo.com

Osteopath Dr. W.O. Faber is a leader in Prolotherapy (reconstructive therapy) that resolves or lessens pain by creating a 30-40% regrowth of ligaments, tendons and joints. www.milwaukeepainclinic.com

Dr. Allen Thomashefsky defines Prolotherapy www.drtom.net/prolotherapy.htm

Dr. Martin Dayton's (Florida) website
www.daytonmedical.com

7.   American Rheumatoid Medical Association

The Arthritis Trust Association links a worldwide association of physicians who specialize in auto-immune or collagen tissue diseases such as osteo or rheumatoid diseases, and many other forms, including Anykylosing Spondelitis (Bamboo Spine).   www.arthritistrust.org

Dr. Milne Ongley's use of Prolotherapy to treat Ankylosing Spondelitis www.ongleyonline.com

8.   International Bio-Oxidative Medical Association
www.bio-proinc.com

What is oxidation? According to the website:

"Most biochemical reactions in the body are balanced through redox mechanisms. Redox means:

(red)uction (ox)idation. Anytime a substance is reduced (chemically changed) something else must be oxidized (chemically changed the other way) for the reactions to stay in balance.

Oxidation, as an example, is the process which causes rust (slow oxidation) or fire (rapid oxidation). In the body, some types of oxidation are thought to be harmful by producing Free Radicals."

Intravenous hydrogen peroxide, hyperbaric oxygen, ozone, anti-oxidant therapy are used as a treatment for many conditions under these disease categories: heart and blood vessel, pulmonary, infectious, immune disorders, and others.

Hyperbaric Medical Association
www.hyperbaricmedicalassociation.org
- Clinics for stroke rehabilitation, parent network for childhood for childhood disorders.

Bio-Immune, Inc.

Clinic resources for immune therapy www.bioimmune.com

E.G., Dr. Naima Abdel Ghany, M.D., Ph.D., Panama City, Florida, uses a multimodality immunotherapy program (MIP). www.bioimmune.com/about_us/investor/press.asp?id=25

9. American Association of Anti-Aging Medicine (A⁴M)

Live longer, healthier. Physicians in 13 countries www.worldhealth.net
Profiles of anti-aging professionals   www.antiaging-systems.com

10. Association for Comprehensive Neuro Therapy

Physician listings for diverse approaches to neurological disorders such as autism, attention deficit disorder/hyperactive, obsessive compulsive, learning disabled, Tourette Syndrome, and delinquency. www.latitudes.org
Chelation treatments/autism www.healing-arts.org/children/main.htm

11. The Cranial Academy

Addresses the cranial aspects of Osteopathy; Cranio-sacral therapy

www.cranialacademy.com

The Academy states:

> "Osteopathic medicine is dedicated to the treatment and healing of the entire patient, rather than approaching a patient's symptoms in a crisis-oriented, one-spot only approach.
>
> This respect for, and study of, the entire functioning of the human system has led to various means of diagnosis and treatment…includes that of manipulation, whereby the physician uses a hands-on approach to assure that the body in moving freely. This free motion ensures that all innate healing systems are free to work unhindered."

(In the section, "What Is Osteopathy?" there is a fascinating description about the primary respiratory mechanism found in all bodies and how these specialists correct its malfunctioning.)

Numerous problems are addressed by cranial osteopaths in these areas, and without drugs/surgery. Areas include pediatrics, systemic, dental problems, orthopedic, genito-urinary, ear/nose/throat, digestive, neurological syndromes, respiratory illness, and pregnancy.

See also:

Upledger Institute, Florida
Dr. John E. Upledger's clinic and educational center www.upledger.com
Dr. Kappel's article, Craniosacral Therapy www.iquestsight.com

12. American College Osteopathic Sclero-therapeutic Pain Medicine Specialists

www.acopms.com/members.htm

13.Chiropractic Specialists

The Gonstead Approach, a directory of chiropractors

www.gonsteadseminar.com
Sacro Occipital Technique (craniopathy) www.sorsi.com
Dr. Frank Painter, info and directory   www.chiro.org
Dr. Goodman, info and directory www.goodmanchiro.com

14. Homeopathic Medicine

"Like cures like and less is more"

Ophthalmologist Dr. Edward Kondrot, M.D., (H), CCH, is a homeopathic ophthalmologist. His website lists homeopathy, micro current stimulation, Chelation therapy, and other alternative treatments for macular degeneration, glaucoma, cataracts, etc. www.homeopathiceye.com Dr. Kondrot defines homeopathy:

"...a scientific method of therapy based on the principle of stimulating the body's own healing processes in order to accomplish cure. The basic system was developed and verified by Samuel Hahnemann, a German physician nearly 200 years ago. Homeopathy's astounding success rates in both chronic and acute diseases has resulted in not only standing the test of time, but rapidly achieving widespread acceptance in Europe, India, and South America.

In Homeopathy (homeo means similar), each of us is a total, complete individual, no aspect of which can be separated from any other. To be effective, any valid therapy must be based on a deep understanding of and respect for the uniqueness of each individual.

In Homeopathy each patient is evaluated as a whole person – mental/emotional/physical. The prescribing remedy is based on the unique patterns found on all three levels. This means that each person is given a remedy that will fit their constitution. Ten people with macular degeneration might receive ten different homeopathic remedies."

Listings of M.D.'s who practice homeopathy
www.homeopathic.org

Internist Dr. Jacob Irman's website
www.demystify.com

A medical homeopathic and nutritional approach
www.alternativemedcare.com

Homeopathic Pharmaceutical Consultants, John Bornemann III, R.
www.homeodrugconsult.com

15. College of Optometrists in Vision Development

www.covd.org

Take charge of your vision with a qualified O.D. trained in behavioral/developmental/rehabilitative optometry. 75% of those who receive in-office, at-home vision therapy (Convergence Insufficiency Treatment) report fewer and less severe symptoms related to reading and other near work. Low tech, safe, simple exercises.

Pro Hockey player Brian Pothier credits this therapy for his recovery from head injury and return to the ice. ESPN NHL News for 03/26/09.

16. American Academy of Medical Acupuncture

Medical doctors who employ acupuncture
www.medicalacupuncture.org

17. American Association of Naturopathic Physicians

The AANP defines Naturopathic Medicine:

> "Naturopathic medicine blends centuries-old natural, non-toxic therapies with current advances in the study of health and human systems, covering all aspects of family health from prenatal to geriatric care...concentrates on whole-patient wellness - the medicine is tailored to the patient and emphases prevention and self-care...attempts to find the underlying cause of the patient's condition rather than focusing solely on symptomatic treatment..."

Find a member doctor: www.naturopathic.org
The Canadian Association of Naturopathic Doctors
www.cand.ca

18. Holistic Dental Association

Complementary and Alternative (metal-free dentistry
www.holisticdental.org
See also Integrative Healthcare Centers of America
www.talkinternational.com

Osteopath Dr. Edward Mercola's dental listings
www.mercola.com
His dentist, Dr. Lina Garcia, DDS/Cranial Osteopath
Fluoride Action Network   www.fluorideaction.net

Formerly in-practice, now researcher Dr. Huggin's website
www.hugnet.com
Books by Dr. Huggins, DDS, MS: _It's All In Your Head (Not)!_

Solving the MS Mystery and Your Goose isn't Cooked Yet!
Elements of Danger: Protect Yourself Against the Hazards of Modern Dentistry
Authors: Morton Walker, D.P.M., and Julian Whitaker, M.D.
www.drmortonwalker.com

Dr. Whitaker on post polio syndrome and many other conditions www.drwhitaker.com world-wide resource to locate holistic/biological health professionals for jawbone cavitations, serum antibody testing for dental material compatibility, amalgam removal, etc.
www.dentalhelp.org

19. Association of Natural Medicine Pharmacists www.anmp.org

Homeopathic Pharmaceutical Consultants, John Bornemann III, R. Ph.
www.homeodrugconsult.com

20. Foundation for the Advancement of Innovative Medicine

FAIM website includes books, tapes and listing of doctors www.faim.org

FAIM board member, Dr. Majid Ali's virtual integrative medical library www.fatigue.net His Institute of Integrative Medicine, NY NJ

Capital University of Integrative Medicine http://www.cuim.edu/
President Dr. Majid Ali, his clinic sites
www.fatigue.net

21. International College of Clinical Medicine

Many chelation doctors belong to this association (formerly The Great Lakes College of Clinical Medicine) www.glccm.org

22. American Holistic Medical Association
www.holisticmedicine.org

23. American Holistic Nurses Asssoociation
www.ahna.org

24. Physician Association for Anthroposophical Medicine
www.paam.net

Offers a holistic, spiritual approach to conventional and alternative medicine

25. International Tibetan Medical Association

Dr. Nyima Namseling's website
www.tibetmed.org

26. International University for Alternative Medicines, Calcutta

Dr. S.K. Agarwal, Pres., Indian Board of Alternative Medicine
www.altmeduniversity.com

27. Physicans   for   Photoluminescence/Blood Irradiation

www.altmedangel.com

28. Insulin Potentiation Therapy   www.getipt.com

Tougher on cancer, etc., – easier on the patient
www.iptforcancer.com

29. Institute for Funtional Medicine

www.functionalmedicine.org

30. Altmeds, a general source for doctors

www.altmeds.com

31. International Academy of Clinical Thermology

www.iact-org.org
Breast thermography for earlier detection

32. Practitioners of Computerized Electro-Dermal Screening

www.cedsdirectory.org

33. Medical Specialists "Galore"

www.bottomlinehealth.com

YOUR NOTES ON MEDICAL ASSOCIATIONS:

Veterinary Medical Associations, for Pets and Service Animals

Locate vets, books, tapes, and other resources for the public. Many members have websites.

1. American Holistic Veterinary Medical Association

www.ahvma.org

2. International Veterinary Acupuncture

www.ivas.org

3. Veterinary Botanical Medical Association

www.vbma.org

4. Academy of Veterinary Homeopathy

www.theavh.org

5. American Veterinary Chiropractic Association

www.animalchiropractic.org

6. Association of Veterinarians for Animal Rights

Realistic alternatives to harming animals in veterinary education and practice; means to avoid heritable, congenital disease in service animals and pets. Founders were V.M.D.'s Neil C. Wolff and Nedim C. Buyukmihci (Be - uke - mah - kah)   www.avar.org

Examples of veterinary alternatives to drugs/surgery:

Orthomolecular Vet, Dr. Wendell Belfield's website with complementary online, bi-monthly web magazine with back issues, all topics in pet health. From a past issue:

> "Idiopathic epilepsy was cured four years ago in an Australian Shepherd who had ten grand mal seizures daily, just by using a skin allergy therapy (essential oils, nutrition) for this central nervous system allergy."

Veterinary Alternative Resources

Extensive information on nutritional approaches to pet healthcare, chronic/acute illnesses, Vitamin C as a remedy for numerous situations.

Dr. Belfield's Nutritional Products and his *How to Have a Healthier Dog*
www.belfield.com

Trauma Vet specialist, Gary M. Tran has observed remarkable results in his trauma/chronic/intractable practice using Tahitian Noni™ (Morinda Citriolic) fruit juice extract. For telephone consultations with Dr. Tran go to www.vetworld.com, Dr. Tran, Louisville, KY.

Noni™ juice has been used successfully to treat West Nile virus in 6 Belgians, 1 Shetland, in Northern Minnesota who were downed from the virus also paralysis in sheep.

For discussion, and books and tapes about results of treatment with Noni™ juice in people and pets observed by Dr. Tran and many other medical doctors; Dr. Tran's audio-tape or physician Neil Solomon's *Noni for Pets* booklet   www.nonitools.com

Michael Fox, DVM

http://tedeboy.tripod.com/drmichaelwfox/id102.html

Dr. Fox is to veterinary medicine as Dr. Hoffer is to orthomolecular medicine: his information is boundless. His recent book is *Not Fit for a Dog - The Truth about Manufactured Dog and Cat Food.*

Veterinarian William Barnett covers health issues in pet food and the desirability for a dog/cat supplement to improve pet health.
Dr. Barnett's nutritional products
www.vetbalance.com

Tumors in Pets – Nutrition for immune enhancement

www.PetAlive.com

See their long list of conditions, including distemper and parvo, treated with homeopathic oral vaccines.

This includes accounts of tumor recession, e.g., a tumor in the nail bed of a Rottweiler. The presiding vet predicted death within a month, so did not recommend amputation.

As the tumor advanced up the front leg, the C-Caps supplement was administered daily and soon the cancer receded and disappeared with no relapse.

Oxygen therapy (hyper-baric oxygen medicine) in veterinary practice
http://hbomedtoday.com/HMT_3/P13.html-9k

You may need to enter or access the above article through
www.hbomedtoday.com , then select Issue 3.

Massage for pets:
www.massageawareness.com

More sources:
Drs. Foster and Smith www.PetEducation.com

Vet-formulated supplements
www.everlifeanimalhealth.com

www.byvetsonly.com

Medical Doctors on pets:
Garry Gordon's website for animal links
www.longevityplus.net
Dr. Stoll's pet section
www.askwaltstollmd.com

YOUR NOTES ON VETS FOR YOUR PETS:

Part 4 – Prominent Treatment Centers and Resources
(Some of many)

International Hospitals for Cancer and Other Chronic Diseases

Patients come from all over the world to these centers which offer complementary medicine (combining traditional and alternative medical approaches). Inquirers feel comfortable seeking information and can contact a physician at no charge.

Insurance should cover 80% costs, as these are accredited hospitals. Most require cash up front, but provide forms for you to submit for reimbursement. For tours of treatment centers in Mexico or the annual Labor Day symposium in the Los Angeles area:
www.cancercontrolsociety.com

NOW IN IRVINE CALIFORNIA - Oasis of Hope Hospital is the hospital of Oncology Surgeon, Francisco Contreras. Oasis uses Fractionated Chemotherapy, a progressive, gradual application administered over longer time periods, 1 to 3 days. Dr. Contreras specialized in surgical oncology at the University Hospital, Vienna, Austria. Oasis offers programs of four days to several weeks duration and now provides the German Issels treatments
www.oasisofhope.com

Twenty years ago, the heir to the Max Factor Corporation, Donald Factor, was healed of stage 4 lung cancer at this hospital. Mr. Factor is featured in a video presentation at this website and shares his recovery from a supposedly incurable stage of cancer. Look for the comparison chart for rates of success in various types of cancer. Don's statistical chances of surviving stage 4 lung cancer were 20% at Contreras, but only 2% with conventional medicine.

Much higher success rates are documented for other cancers. Oasis Hospital plans expansions to England and S. Korea. Currently, patients come from all over the industrialized world to be treated by the Contreras Medical Family and their staff.

In a recent case, two elderly sisters flew from Denmark to Mexico (27 hours with four flight changes) to be treated at Oasis Hospital. A physician from Saudi Arabia avowed that Oasis is the only hospital he would consider for his father's cancer treatment. On arrival, a Canadian could hardly walk through the door, but a few weeks later strode out after completing his treatment, carrying his own heavy suitcase. Not everyone can make it, but statistically speaking, more recover here using an integrative approach of conventional and non-conventional medicine than with conventional only, especially in cases where the cancer has spread. Whatever you choose, the early bird gets the worm.

During the Summer, 2009, regarding the Minnesota runaway mother with son, on Larry King, Dr. Contreras acknowledged the need for fractionated (slow dose) chemotherapy in the treatment of Hodgkins in conjunction with immune and nutritional support. See also Cancer Treatment Centers for fractionated chemo.

The legacy of Dr. Josef Issels, another German protocol, continues on the top floor of the Oasis Hospital. Observe photos of before/after cases of supposedly incurable cancer. www.issels.org

International Bio Care Hospital and Medical Center (IBC Hospital)
Medical Director, Dr. Rodrigo Rodriquez
www.ibchospital.com

St. Joseph Hospital – Across from Brownsville, Texas
www.doctorofhope.com

Directed by Oncologist, Charles Rogers, M.D., Cherokee Nation of Mexico

Descriptions of various cancers: this doctor's innovations in drugless approaches; testimonials, recovery from advanced stages involving difficult types of cancer.

The Pomeranian Academy of Medicine, Poland

Offers spas, medical fasting centers all over the world
http://www.ams.edu.pl/

Dr. Peter Wolf's Hannover Clinic
www.hyperthermia-centre-hannover.com
ITP (Insulin Potentiated Treatment) and Fever Therapy for cancer–

Dr. Nieper's work continues with German Dr. med. Peter Wolf.

Multiple Sclerosis:

–German legacy of Hans Nieper, M.D., U.S. Source

www.mwt.net/~drbrewer/

–Dr. Joachim Ledwoch - Continues the work of Dr. Nieper
www.dr-ledwoch.de

-Dr. Nieper's Calcium Orotate

www.naturalhealthconsult.com/Monographs/calEAP.html

ITL – Immuno-Technologies Cancer Clinic, Freeport Bahamas
www.ImmuneMedicine.com

Emphasis on cancer vaccines, therapies involve Immuno-Augmentive, Heat Shock Protein, Dendritic Cell, also Cytokines and Cachexia Vaccinie to help prevent wasting syndrome.

English physician, Dr. John Clement, is the medical director. Testimonials of advanced recoveries.

UNITED STATES:

Oasis of Hope (Contreras Hospital) now in Irvine Calaifornia
www.cfnmedicine.com

Black Hills Health and Education Center   www.bhhec.org
Located minutes from the Black Hills of South Dakota, this is a month-long medical wellness and lifestyle program.

The Gerson Institute
Provides a wealth of information in its latest book, *Healing Cancer through Diet*   www.gerson.org

Bradford Research Institute (BRI)
www.bradfordresearchinstitute.com

Cancer Treatment Centers of America
www.cancercenter.com
Illinois, Pennsylvania, Tulsa, now the Phoenix area. Other centers are listed, including conventional, also one that employs alternatives for advanced cases. Testimonials for recovery from gastro-esophageal can-

cer, etc. "Patient Empowered Medicine," including fractionated (slowly infused over longer time period) chemotherapy.

Envita Medical Centers of Scottsdale, Arizona
www.envita.com
A clinic for reversal of Cancer, Auto-immune, other chronic diseases. Read patient before/after testimonials for recovery from supposedly incurable stages in cancer, also recovery from Valley Fever.

Hippocrates Institute-headquarters in West Palm, Florida
www.hippocratesinst.org For natural food/supplement healing.

German New Medicine in Nevada www.renointegrative.com
Dr. Brodie's legacy continues.

Dr. Lorraine Day, former Orthopedic Surgeon
http://www.drday.com
Resources from a formerly "terminal" breast cancer patient

Emil Schandle, Ph.D., Hollywood Florida www.CAProfile.com
For earlier cancer detection, 10-12 years in advance is now possible, combined with a pro-active health restoration to balance body chemistry with participating doctors throughout the U.S.

Further resources for selecting a treatment center, some of which charge a fee:

www.alternativemedicine.com California founder, Burton Goldberg
www.beatcancer.org Pennsylvania founder, Susan Silberstein, Ph.D.
www.cancercontrolsociety.com Los Angeles founder, Lorraine Rosenthal
www.canhelp.com Washington founder, Patrick McGrady
www.mnwelldir.org   Minnesota-based
www.mossreport.com New York founder, Robert Moss, Ph.D.
www.cancerdecisions.com
www.peopleagainstcancer.com Iowa founder,   Frank Wiewel
www.naturalcancertherapies.com
www.cancer-central.com Resources on the effectiveness of a liquid, Tian Xian Free PDF, "The Cancer Terminator, 100 Survival testimonies.

NOTE: Insurance does not cover <u>clinic</u> care as readily as <u>hospital</u> care.
There are more cancer clinics listed in the Cancer Section of Part 5, Diseases/Conditions.

Part 5 – Examples of Disease or Condition

"If you still have five minutes of lucid thought process, your Alzheimer's is reversible."

– Dr. Abram Hoffer, MD, PhD, Orthomolecular Psychiatrist from

Beating Alzheimer's

By recovered Alzheimer's patient, Tom Warren
Mr. Warren used to have an impressive, 30 page website. Order his book through Amazon.

A quick reference guide online
www.askwaltstollmd.com
A glossary of treatments for conditions
www.daytonmedical.com

Dr. Balch's tomé, *Prescription for Nutritional Healing* **3ʳᵈ Ed.**
www.amazon.com

An in-depth publication on supplements, foods for 250 conditions

Alternative Medicine - The Definitive Guide, **2002**
www.alternativemedicine.com

An in-depth publication on numerous treatments, resources

Most of the doctors in the following websites treat a variety of conditions. For example, the following are addressed at Dr. Jonathan Wright's clinic (see also his www.meridianvalleylab.com) in Tahoma, Washington:

Allergy, arthritis, asthma, atherosclerosis, auto immune disorders, bursitis, colitis, cancer, depression, diabetes, digestive disorders, fatigue, fibromyalgia, glaucoma, headaches, high blood pressure, cholesterol, macular degeneration, natural hormone replacement for men/women, osteoporosis, overweight, recurrent infections, shingles, and women's health issues.

Alcoholism
-Metabolic restoration
www.healthrecovery.com

Alzheimer's, Organic Brain Syndromes
Dr. Cranton's website
www.drcranton.com

"If you still have five minutes of lucid thought process, your Alzheimer's is reversible."

– Dr. Abram Hoffer, MD, PhD, Orthomolecular Psychiatrist from *Beating Alzheimer's* - recovered Alzheimer's patient, Tom Warren's book. (Mr. Warren used to have a 30 page, scientific website:

www.midnightcafe.com/alzh/)

Florida Neurologist Dr. David Perlmutter's clinic and book, *Brain Recovery,* also his success in reversing Parkinson's.   www.perlhealth.com

Dr. Wright's clinic (with Japanese and Spanish translations)

www.tahoma-clinic.com

Toxic Metal Syndrome: How Metal Poisoning Can Affect Your Brain
By H.R. Casdorph, MD, PhD, and Morton Walker, DPM.
www.acam.org
www.drmortonwalker.com

Defense against Alzheimer's by H.J. Roberts, MD
(see also his book under Diabetes)
www.sunsentpress.com

AIDS – Acquired Immune Deficiency Syndrome
California physician Jon D. Kaiser's 15+ years success in AIDS recovery; his clinic, phone and e-mail consultation service and books.
www.jonkaiser.com

Dr. Kaiser's book,
Healing HIV and Immune Power: The Comprehensive Healing Program for HIV
Burton Goldberg Group,
You Don't Have To Die
www.alternativemedicine.com

Australian Dr. Ian Brighthope's book, *The AIDS Fighters: The Role of Vitamin C & Other Immunity-Building Nutrients*, Keats Publishing www.amazon.com

Description of Dr. Brighthope's book:
www.cqs.com/aidscure.htm

"I have yet to lose a full blown AIDS patient who stuck to my vitamin C protocol." - **Dr. Brighthope**

This doctor has been associated with the following Australian Medical Assn. www.acnem.org

Dr. Cathcart's website   www.orthomed.org

Allergy, Asthma, ADHD
Dr. Mary Ann Block's Dallas area clinic

www.blockcenter.com

Dr. Keith Scott-Mumby's *Food Allergy Plan* and *The Complete Guide to Food Allergy and* Environmental Illness.

www.alternativedoctor.com

www.aaem.org

www.acam.org

www.orthomed.org

Over-the-counter: www.nonitestimonials.com

ALS Amyotrophic Lateral Sclerosis
(muscular degeneration)

www.orthomed.org

In Vienna, Austria, for ALS
www.kroisscancercenter.com

Check the Mexican complementary medicine facilities

www.cancercontrolsociety.com

San Diego Clinic (also for Multiple Sclerosis)

www.sdclinic.com

Ankylosing Spondelites ("Bamboo Spine")
Prolotherapy physician, Dr. Milne Ongley's website
www.ongleyonline.com

Anthrax (vitamin C as a proposed adjuvant) **also
Hemorrhagic Fevers: Dengue, Ebola, etc.**
www.orthomed.com
Dr. Day on Anthrax   www.drday.com

Aspartame Disease? Birth Defects see also Diabetes
Complications of Aspartame are thoroughly described by internist of
Palm Springs Florida., H.J. Robertson in his hilarious *Sweet'ner Dearest,
and* other publications www.sunsentpress.com

HHS 1994, submission of 92 reported symptoms submitted to the FDA
for potential side-effects

Neurosurgeon, Dr. Russell Blaylock
www.aspartamekills.com

Autism – see good results with I.V. Chelation.
www.dorway.com
National listing of doctors by state who chelate children with autism to
remove mercury
www.healing-arts.org/children/amyholmes.htm

Google "troublemakers" Dr. Jerry Kartzinel, actress Jenny McCarthy for
an exponential resource!

Brain Recovery:

Dr. Perlmutter's website: www.brainrecovery.com
Dr. Psy. Daniel Amen' www.amenclinics.com
Neurosurgeon Russell Blaylock... google "All things Blaylock"

Find **ALTERNATIVE** M.D.s

More Cancer Clinics/Centers:
All over the world, plus other conditions
www.cancure.org
Cancer Clinics/Centers in Europe:

Bristol Cancer Help Centre of England
www.bristolcancerhelp.org

Kroiss Cancer Center, Vienna, Austria
www.kroisscancercenter.com

Dr. Nieper's legacy continues in Germany
www.dr-ledwoch.de

St. Georgi Klinik, Bad Abling, Southern Germany
www.klinik-st-georg.de

Oncology, immunology, and environmental research of Dr. Helmut Keller.
For many other sites on specific types of cancer.
www.cancer2000.com

Lukas Klinik, Switzerland
www.lukasklinik.ch

More Cancer Clinics/Centers in North America:

Dr. Emil Schandl's earliest possible detection 10-12 years in advance

www.CAprofile.net

Reputable resources

www.cancercontrolsociety.com
www.cancerdecisions.com   www.mossreport.com
www.canhelp.com
www.naturalcancertherapies.com

Hoffer's Home page "Orthomolecular Treatment of Cancer"

www.islandnet.com/~hoffer/   If not available try:

www.doctoryourself.com

Dr. Charles Roger's St. Joseph Hospital Clinic, across from Brownsville, Texas Descriptions of various cancers, testimonials of advanced recoveries

www.doctorofhope.com

International Clinic for Biological Rejuvenation
—Cell therapy clinics in England, Nassau, and Mexico
www.icbr.com

—European live cell (shark embryo) therapy
www.extendlilfe.com

—Cell specific cancer therapy, Europe, Dom. Rep
www.csct.com

Immuno-Augmentative Therapy Clinic, Bahamas
www.immunemedicine.com

Internist Naima Abdel-Ghany's Florida Clin
www.bioimmune.com

Internist Keith Block, Evanston, Illinois
www.blockmd.com

Dr. Nick Gonzales, Park Avenue, New York Clinic, - interviewed on public Television; also on Larry King with Dr. Burzynski - Fall, 2009 along with Suzanne Sommer's book entitled "Knockout."

www.dr-gonzales.com

Dr. Privatera's California clinic. Diagnosis with dark field microscopy
www.nutriscreen.com

Houston Doctor. Stanislaw Burzynski's Anti-Neoplaston Therapy
www.cancermed.com
See a variety of successful reversals, including many childhood brain
related tumors

Learn about bio-electrotherapy (BET), used clinically in Europe and
China for more than 100 years.
www.newhopeclinic.com

"The Cancer Personality," German New Medicine, etc. – Dr. Brodie's
Nevada clinic
www.drbrodie.com/personality.html

Cancer: The Definitive Guide is a major volume featuring medical experts
and their nontoxic approaches to cancer.
Published by Burton Goldberg Group.
Order from www.alternativemedicine.com, a monthly magazine that
features helpful advertising from the growing number of reputable clinics, hospitals who employ alternatives to drugs and surgery.

Cardiovascular
See also Part 3 - Medical Associations #1 and #2.
Fascinating before/after pictures of Dr. Hohnbaum's feet in Dr. Walker's
classic, _Everything You Should know About Chelation._
See this on www.amazon.com or purchase the book with pictures
from Amazon or www.drmortonwalker.com.

–Impressive info on heart disease and recovery:
www.gordonresearch.com and google
"All things Dean Ornish, M.D. or go to
www.pmri.org.

–Dr. West's approach to Congestive Heart Failure (CHF)
www.mnwelldir.org/docs/cardio15.htm

–Inflammation, cardiology's newest frontier
www.myheartbook.com

–Over-the-counter, Dr. Gordon endorses Norwegian fish oil on TV
www.icelandhealth.com
–Over-the-counter, Rice bran formula for cardiovascular health
www.tryricenshine.com

Chemical Nerve Agents and Poisons – See Gulf War Vets

Children/Adults, numerous conditions of:
ADHD, allergy, asthma, autism, etc. www.alternative-mentalhealth.com

MUMS, a national parent to parent support ne
www.hbotofaz.org
Inquire for child medical care from medical associations, ACAM, AAEM, ISOM

Congestive Heart Disease – Dr. West's approach
www.mnwelldir.org/docs/cardio15.htm

Developmental Delay (retardation and Downs Syndrome for infant/children) Refer to Dr. Leigh's discussion in Part I, and Part 2, also www.kospublishing.com

Downs Syndrome and Cognitive Delay – For a dramatic and typical healing, pictures show normalization of a little girl with Down's

(Dr. Schmidt); also the before/after pictures of a six year old boy with retardation and his IQ improvement from 50 to 90 using live cell injections, in

Dr. Kühnau's *Live-Cell Therapy*, page 123 (out of print). Request edition that contains the pictures

Diabetes, see also Thyroid/Endocrine

Dr. Gabriel Cousens's Arizona clinic for natural recovery from diabetes
www.treeoflife.nu/diabetes

Aspartame - 92 conditions documented by the FDA related to consumption of aspartame, a dietary sugar replacement; also 16 diseases that aspartame mimics or aggravates.

Florida Internist H.J. Roberts, M.D., F.A.C.P., F.C.C.P. Books and tapes about artificial sweeteners, other medical issues, including *Aspartame Disease: An Ignored Epidemic, Sweet'ner Dearest*
www.sunsentpress.com

"Emerging Facts About Aspartame"
(Journal, Diabetic Association of India 1995: Vol. 35, 4
Dr. J. Barua, Ophth., Surgeon A.Bal.
www.dorway.com/barua.html

For Diabetic Peripheral Neuropathy
www.tahoma-clinic.com

Endometriosis
www.endometriosisassn.org

Eyes – glaucoma, macular, cataract, etc.
Ophthalmologist Edward Kondrot
www.homeopathiceye.com

Optometrist Garry Kappel, O.D., F.C.V.O.D.
www.iquestsight.com

College of Optometrists in Vision Development
www.covd.org

Dr. Gary Price Todd (deceas). Google for his books, e.g., _Smart Medicine For Your Eyes._

M.D. Jonathan Wright's clinic
www.tahomaclinic.com

The Cambridge Institute for Better Vision
www.bettervision.com

Find an alternative doctor for eye care
www.visionworksusa.com

Fatigue (CFIDS)
Beyond the Dark Cloud: Road to Recovery from Chronic Fatigue and Immune System Dysfunction
–by Thea Schlossner, foreword by Jay Goldstein, M.D., The author's website: www.smallbusinesses.com/schlosse.htm

Gender Specific Conditions and the "eight little culprits" that cause it.

Both genders are entitled to adequate levels of hormone for balance. The eight involved glands are: adrenal, pituitary, ovaries, testes, thyroid, para-thyroid, pancreas, pineal. Issues include male andropause/female menopause, impotence, infertility, low sex drive, cancers, etc.

Dr. Barnes' medical foundation for thorough diagnosis of thyroid function – lab samples sent to Belgium.
www.brodabarnes.org

Tissue Mineral (hair) Analysis to determine hormone levels
www.meltdown.com
www.hormoneprofile.com

(Over-the-counter) Improve progesterone, testosterone balance
www.zellersnaturalhealth.com
Also available, saliva testing for hormonal balance.

Maximizing Manhood: Beating the Male Menopause
by Malcolm Carruthers, M.D., London.
Testosterone deficiencies in men; support groups for women.
www.brodabarnes.com

Sexual Enhancement,
By Dr. Graham Simpson
www.agelesszonereno.com
Erectile Disfunction
Address the cause (it may be nutritional deprivation) without drugs
Park Avenue Chelation physician, Mike Tepliskey's super libido and super prostate formulas
www.physicianschoice.net

MEDICARE-endorsed: Posty-vak's three safe approaches to E.D.
www.rejoyn.com

Gynecologist Helen Penanti's natural solutions for middle-age needs
Grateful husbands, relieved wives from her topical/insertion formulas
www.askdrhelen.com

Natural alternatives to synthetic hormone replacement therapy
www.johnrlee.com See also, Thyroid

GERD Gastric Esophageal Reflex Syndrome (see Indigestion)
Gastric By-Pass Surgeon Gary Snyder's alternative to his own surgery

www.fullbar.com

Gulf War Syndrome,
Military nurse Joyce Riley (ret) advocacy
www.gulfwarvets.com

Aspartame, especially if consumption at high temperature
www.aspartamekills.com

Agent Orange effects from Vietnam
Sub-lingual Vitamin B12 (methyl-cobalamin injections) for Peripheral Neuropathy.
A Vietnam veteran immediately recovers from tremors, just with B-12 lozenges, (sub-lingual)

www.buzzle.com/articles/alternative-treatment-for-peripheral-neuropathy-agent-orange

Dr. Libby's discovery of sublingual vitamin B complex
www.sublingualb12.com
An Environmentally triggered illness
www.aaem.com
Dr. Huggins' site for Environmental Illness (E.I.)
www.hugnet.com

Heart, See also Cardio-vascular
www.paulingtherapy.com
www.icelandhealth.com
www.thecureforheartdisease.com

Heavy Metals, Removal of
www.meltdown.com/metals.htm
www.ironoverload.org

Hepatitis
Dr. Cathcart's website
www.orthomed.com
International Society for Orthomolecular Medicine (ISOM)
www.orthomed.org

Liver health information, Dr. Cabot's website
www.liverdoctor.com
Extensive resources, Hepatitis C
www.objectivemedicine.com

Huntington's Chorea
–Dr. Hoffer's success in controlling Huntington's with essential fatty acids can be found in *Townsend Letter for Doctors,* order March, 1997.
www.tldp.com
–At Dr. Velasquez site, ask for Phillip Hardt
www.extendlife.com

IBS (Irritable Bowel Syndrome) see Indigestion

Immune Therapy
Clinic directory for Bioimmune Inc.
www.bioimmune.com

Indigestion!
A Duluth doctor "to the rescue"
www.mnmed.org/publications/
Over-the-counter:
www.aloecurerelief.com www.colocerin.com www.myseaaloe.com

Infertility – Dr. Yvonne Scott-Miller's approach
www.dryvonnescottmiller.com

Iron Overload Diseases Association
www.ironoverload.org

Liver problems, see Hepatitis

Lupus
Dr. Wright's clinic
www.tahoma-clinic.com

Lyme's Disease
Drs. J.W. Forsythe, M.D., H.M.D. and K.C. Tang, M.D., H.M.D.

Many other chronic conditions, treated including cancer.
www.centurywellness.com

Canadian Lymes' Disease
www.canadianlymediseasefoundation.org
Pet, People, and Lymes'
www.canlyme.com

Mental Health
Clinical Nutritionist, Carol Simontachi's
The Crazy Makers – How the Food Industry is Destroying Our Brains and Harming Our Children.
A helpful synopsis of her December 29, 2008 radio interview is available at www.coasttocoastam.com under past shows. Effects from chlorine, fluoride, and other chemicals are also addressed.

Multiple Sclerosis
Neurologist David Perlmutter, Naples, Florida Clinic
www.perlhealth.com

Dr. Huggins' *Solving The MS Mystery: Recovery, Auto-Immune Disease*
www.hugnet.com

Pain in Joints
See Part 3 - Medical Associations - sections on Orthopedic, Rheumatoid, Chiropractic, Osteopathy, Craniopathy. To avoid most joint surgery, see Part 6, Appendix 3.

Parkinson's – use of Glutathione for
Dr. Ronald Hoffman's Park Avenue clinic
www.drhoffman.com
Dr. Perlmutter's Florida clinic
www.perlhealth.com

Post-Polio Syndrome, go to Dr. Whitaker, click on Wellness, Inc.
www.drwhitaker.com

Prostate (BHP, cancer)
New York physician Michael Schachter's clinic, book on the prostate
www.mbschachter.com
Dr. Friedrich Douwes' book and prostate clinic
www.klinik-st-georg.de

Reputable capsule, often oil-based formulas exist for BHP normalization within days to a month:
Dr. Tepliskey's Super Prostrate:
www.physicianschoice.net
Dr. Garry Gordon's Prostrate Contro
www.icelandhealth.com

Structural - Bad Back, Limbs, etc.
See Orthopedic, Arthritis, Chiropractic specialties in File 3 – Medical Associations.
For neurological complications, in Minneapolis area
www.officialsynapse.com

Systemic Lupus Erythematosis (SLE)
Systemic Lupus Erythemtosis by Jean Pierog, R.N., M.S.
www.healthlinks.net/archive/lupus.html

Thyroid Conditions and Diseases - See also Gender
"Health begins and ends with the proper balance of the endocrine system."
Dr. Broda Barnes, M.D.

Dr. Barnes (deceased) has written *Hypo-Thyroidism: The Hidden Illness*
Research Foundation
www.brodabarnes.org

"Top Doctor Lists" for alternative thyroid care in the United States and 15 other countries.
www.thyroid.about.com/cs/doctors
www.wilsonssyndrome.com

Toxic Metal Syndrome
Toxic Metal Syndrome: How Metal Poisoning Can Affect Your Brain by H.R. Casdorph, M.D., Ph.D., chelation doctor; and Morton Walker, DPM, monthly columnist in *The Townsend Letters*.

Detailed but readable accounts of recoveries from Alzheimer's, and other organic brain recoveries, by removal of toxic (heavy) metals via I.V. chelation, and other antioxidant methods. To order on-line at www.acam.org or www.drmortonwalker.com

Vaccination Side Effects
National Vaccine Information Center
www.909shot.com

Vertigo, dizziness, imbalance, see Vestibular

Vestibular - inner-ear balance disorders. Acoustic neuronal, benign paroxysmal positional vertigo (BPPB), Meniere's, labyrinthitis.

VEDA, The Vestibular Disorders Association, "Symptoms of vestibular disorder may include dizziness, imbalance, vertigo, nausea, and fuzzy vision and may be accompanied by hearing problems."
www.vestibular.org

Vision – See Eyes

Yeast Syndrome – affects men, women, and children.
A systemic problem, yeast can affect both genders, and all ages. Inquire of doctors in ACAM, AAEM, ISOM, and other medical associations. Dr William Crook's www.yeastconnection.com is an established resource.

Remember:

Do your homework for prices, ingredients, strength variations, etc., when buying "over the counter."

Also, the authors have no vested interests in any such products, clinics, doctors, etc.

YOUR NOTES:

Part 6 – Appendices

Appendix 1. Insurance Coverage

Alternative Health Insurance Services of California
www.alternativeinsurance.com

Group and individual policies allow freedom of choice for alternative and conventional methods.

"Alternative and complementary medical benefits are now available to businesses and individuals through integrative health plans designed and negotiated by Alternative Health Insurance Services."

CareCredit®
www.CareCredit.com

Your doctor must be a participator for this (initially) no interest, monthly payment plan.

For example, Prolotherapy specialist, Dr. Mark Wheaton, is a participating doctor.

A minimal amount is due monthly at no interest, unless payments are late.

CAUTION: INTEREST INCREASES SIGNIFICANTLY AFTER THE GRACE PERIOD SO PLAN AHEAD

MEDICARE
Finally, Medicare covers I.V. Chelation Therapy in the states of Delaware, Maryland, West Virginia, and Washington.

Appendix 2. A Perspective on Supplements by Dr. Leigh

In my own practice I provided superior supplements as a convenience to my patients. It is important to have a basic knowledge of the relative importance of the nutrients and of the dosages listed on the items under consideration. Also helpful are the synergized multivitamin, mineral formulas. There are countless other sound formulas, but investigate carefully.

Here are some general guidelines that I provided for my patients to give a basic understanding of what to expect from nutritional supplementation:

1. Our bodies are self-healing.

2. Drugs are useful toxins that, when used properly and for short periods, can shorten illness by allowing our immune systems to kick in.

3. Nutrition is the sum of the vitamins, minerals and energy producing foods we need in order to function

4. Nutritional therapy is the clinical modulation of essential nutrients to augment our immune systems.

5. Antioxidant therapy is designed to prevent damage to our tissues from uncontrolled oxidation.

6. Oxidation is the chemical reaction that makes us warm blooded, and provides the energy to make our bodies run.

Health is the result of the sum of our nutrition, and the control of nature's oxidation   chemistry.

7. There is no single nutrient that will solve all of our health problems.

8. If supplements fail to maintain health, seek professional medical advice.

9. It's much cheaper to stay healthy than to get well!

Related Sources:
For medically authored books on dieting
www.brodabarnes.org

For information on supplements/conditions, etc.
www.drweil.com

How to feed yourself,
Food Preparation: Hints on Making It Happen
www.iquestsight.com

Dr. Huggins' *Your Goose Isn't Cooked Yet!*
www.hugnet.com

Appendix 3. Television and Radio Resources

Reputable Medical and Nutritional Information on TV (yes, TV).
Watch for:

–Dr. Garry Gordon's infomercials for a number of conditions.
www.icelandhealth.com

–Former FDA attorney, Andrew Lessman offers scientifically backed information on the value of supplementation from numerous medical journals, e.g., Journal of Geriatric Psychiatry, Journal of Food Science.

Lessman appears tri-monthly, weekend appearances on Cable HSN, April/July/October/January. Informative presentations on the quality level and amount in supplements; how supplements rarely need fillers, binders of any kind (corn, soy, etc.)   www.pro-caps.com

–Internist Dr. Larry May's endorsement of Prosvent for relief from BHP   www.prosvent.com

–Listen for alternative doctors and researchers on www.coasttocoastam.com   radio, a dignified interview format; respected hosts are George Noory on weeknights, and Ian Punnet weekends. Serious investigative reporters, authors and progressive physicians (e.g., medical leaders on Morgellon's) are featured and allowed to speak out on this late night show. If you are new to the program, don't be dissuaded by certain other topics. This well-received program will soon be televised. Get a load of May 15, 2010's www.responsibletechnology.org for emerging medical discoveries against Genetically Modified foods.

–From TBN, The Trinity Broadcasting Company:
Fascinating presentations on successful, drugless management of numerous health subjects.

Mostly MD's, some ND'S and dentists are featured on programs such as "Ask the Doctor," "Doctor to Doctor," "Biblical Health Moment," Dr. Saxion's "Alternative Health" currently Tuesdays 10 a.m. to 12 p.m. CST, with evening repeat.

Programs replay for a period of time; new doctors and presentations follow. Sample "icons" are:

– Jordan Rubin, NMD. Ph.D., All-encompassing Biblical Health Institute www.jordanrubin.com
Recovered from poor health himself, he is a published leader on nutrition for cancer and other conditions. Watch for his hands-on bus tour presentations www.perfectweightamerica.com

-Dr. Valerie Saxion, N.D.
www.valeriesaxion.com
Dr. Saxion recently described effective, inexpensive, non-drug approaches to depression; on another program she acknowledged the value of suppository chelation for the removal of mercury in the body, as well as biological dentistry. Both of these doctors have warm, engaging personalities, and are hilarious in their own ways.

–NBC's www.DrOz.com **and** www.askthedoctors.com are bridging the gap between conventional and alternative medicine.

Appendix 4. Conditions Treated with Embryonic Cell Transplant Therapy

Courtesy of Thea Schlosser, on behalf of Dr. Kühnau, from his book, _My Life with Live Cell Therapy_:

"My own 41 years' experience with cellular or live cell therapy and that of other researchers has confirmed its great utility in a vast array of conditions and challenges, including but not necessarily limited to:

Chronic arthritis
Chronic pancreatitis
Arteriosclerosis
Liver sclerosis
Allergies of all kinds, except perhaps asthma
Genetic disorders, dysfunctions and physical disturbances
Sexual disorders including impotence
Mental retardation, Down 's syndrome
Chronic lung disease
Chronic kidney disease
Eye disease

Neurological disorders, including epilepsy, multiple sclerosis, Alzheimer's disease, ALS, Parkinson's, post-stroke paralysis, hormone-dependent dysfunctions including sexual disorders Obesity, adrenal insufficiency, hypo-thyroidism.

Hereditary developmental abnormalities of bone and cartilage including dwarfism, congenital hip malformations, congenital dysplasias, spinal problems, cleft palate; cranial and other head malformations (of course, in collaboration with a plastic surgeon)

Muscular dystrophy
Auto-immune diseases in general
Narcolepsy
Rejuvenation
Cancer"

(See separate commentary on cancer in Dr. Kühnau's book. Currently out-of-print, try ordering from Amazon.

For further medical information on live cell and related approaches:

www.extendlife.com
http://spinal.siteutopia.net

Appendix 5. Fix Your Joint Injury with "Prolo" Shots

Sports/Work/Military/Auto

Joint injury (of the connective tissues ligament, tendon, cartilage) can be fixed without drugs/surgery.

Meds who fix them can be located by state at
www.getprolo.com.
Only auto insurance and Workman's Comp cover the injections.

See www.CareCredit.com for an interest-free payment plan for participating doctors – Minnesota's Dr. Mark Wheaton is a participating doctor.

Prolotherapy Injections (to proliferate atrophied cells) is endorsed by the ACC, Atlantic Coast Conference. It is not a banned substance and prolo doctors avoid cortisone injections. The authors prepared the following for Minnesota coaches, but it is useful for coaches elsewhere:

For the Coach

College athletes at Virginia Tech, The Hokies, receive on-campus, Prolotherapy injections from the department head and head team physician, Dr. Gunnar Brolinson. He is pictured injecting the knee of a woman trackster in the June, 2005 track feature
www.theacc.com.

Minnesota coaches/athletes are the last to learn of this FDA-approved, medically verified, non-surgical approach to healing all forms of sports joint injury to the ligament, tendon, cartilage.

Find **ALTERNATIVE** M.D.s

Effective for athletes through all stages of life:

—From the gifted, early athlete who stretches out connective tissue before his/her senior year

—College play

—Professional players – note the websites on the next page.

—Even post competition and coaches (who would appreciate daily routines without agony, comfortable exercise) can shore up their loose (tensile overload), painful joints.

'Iron Man' Ross Hauser, M.D., explains the detrimental effect of icing a joint (as opposed to a muscle) injury and the improvement that M.E.A.T. (movement, exercise, analgesics, prolo treatment) has over R.I.C.E. www.caringmedical.com Look up his
"Sports Injuries: M.E.A.T.—Why we recommend it." Dr. Hauser's second website is www.chicagosportsmedicine.com.

In Excelsior, Minnesota, sports medicine specialist, Dr. Mark Wheaton www.drmarkwheaton.com conducts a monthly Friday/Saturday clinic, third weekend every month in Menahga, ten miles south of Park Rapids www.naturalealternatives.com. Dr. Wheaton explained the medical veracity of Prolotherapy on ESPN's "Outside the Line" after the outcry from stuffed shirts on the Olympic Committee upon hearing that four U.S. Olympic skiers received the injections.

Note that this clinic is owned by Ernest Huttah, prominent muscle and massage therapist who employs a variety of listed manual, and some equipment methods for rehabilitation. Area high school athletes, non-athletes take advantage of his skill from all over Northern Minnesota.

In Minnetonka, featured on WCCO News last year, is Dr. John Odom who is not listed   in getprolo.com but is involved with MN State H.S. Sports)   www.odomsports.com.

In Bloomington, and Minnetonka, there is Dr. Kramer
www.georgekramermd.com

In Blaine, Dr. Mark Janiga
www.janigaprolotherapy.com

In Wisconsin, Dr. William Faber
www.milwaukeepainclinic.com

Other Prolo Docs with good masters/doctoral subject material:

Dr. Ross Hauser, Chicago: www.chicagosportsmedicine.com and www.caringmedical.com and his text, _Prolo Your Sports Injuries Away_ , nearly 1,000 pages in-depth A-Z sports/injuries, in which one orthopedic surgeon states that he has reduced his knee replacement operations by 80%.

Eagles middle linebacker Mark Simoneau, Oakland Raider's Mike Carey tower over Dr.Greenberg, smiling after their shots (current website may no longer carry this photo).Using www.getprolo.com go to PA, So. New Jersey/Phillie area or www.prolotherapy-md.com.

Dr. Marc Darrow, M.D., J.D., Los Angeles: www.jointrehab.com View Detroit tight-end, Jerry Sloan's injection for severe turf toe, and wide receiver Johnny Morton for a thumb injury which healed after only two injections, two weeks apart giving him his first pain-free football season in years.

Click on READ MORE, then find "Muscle and Fitness" magazine, click on picture of the girl feeling the athlete's muscles.

For significant medical material:
www.valleysports.com
Click on Prolotherapy.

These doctors are well-linked with much repetition, but many have different material. Their non-surgical approach is making steady progress toward the mainstream and is an excellent subject area for graduate papers. The medical information and helpful doctors are easily accessed online or in person, as Prolotherapy fortunately lacks the political controversy found in other areas of alternative medicine.

Not all athletes get eliminated from their career paths from connective tissue injury, but for those who do, Prolotherapy can usually rehabilitate a sports career, even improve upon it. Pro athletes sometimes aim for a quadrupling of tendon strength and a doubling of tendon size (Hauser) for example. Of course, the early bird gets the worm.

Any concerns you may have for "interfering," in particular with a public school athlete, may be eased with your role as an informed resource. To treat or not to, is always a decision between parent and doctor anyway. Considering the favorable, trusted relationship that usually exists between coach, parent, athlete, this need not be a problem.

The temporary interest-free payment plan through www.CareCredit.com can make the difference in affordability. One gifted high school athlete's multiple injuries totaled about $7,000. but most athletic injuries are fewer in number.

The authors have developed a simple, easy to apply narrative script that student athletes could act out for themselves with a camcorder. This has good fund raising potential for the right situation. Contact the authors' book response e-mail address if you may be interested.

For the athlete in need of a science, health, even social studies paper or discussion topic, the enclosed sources are easy to access and process.

A final source, in the rare event of a paralyzing injury, a reputable treatment center has success in reversing paralysis, providing the spinal cord is not severed and at least one-fourth of the spinal matrix remains intact. Cost several years ago was approximately $69,000 which includes much follow-up. http://spinal.siteutopia.net

An unrelated alternative info source for men, baseball's Phil Garner is a spokesman and three year consumer of a prostate formula, "Super Beta Prostate" (stilbesterol or plant-based) www.newvitality.com, Numerous other over-the-counter formulas exist, some are listed in Part 5, Conditions/Diseases.

The following letter was published in *The Pioneer* Newspaper, Bemidji, MN, 04/16/06 by Ms. Hagberg and Dr. Leigh.
(Parents and student athletes may find interesting research topics throughout Appendix 5).

"Local Athletes Find Success in Surgery-free Joint Protocol"

"As the agony and ecstasy of high school basketball subsides, off-season is the ideal time for parents of injured players to examine a safe, effective medical option for sports joint (connective tissue) injury.

Park Rapids area parents are taking advantage of the monthly (drug free, no banned substance) injection clinic by elite sports medicine specialist Dr. Mark Wheaton, whose main clinic is located in Excelsior on Minnetonka Bay. He has volunteered as team doctor for Orono footballers and other Twin City sports programs.

AMA endorsed in the 1950s, reconstructive injection therapy or Prolotherapy (for proliferation of one's own cells to re-grow joint tissue) this problem solver is available as close as Menahga.

A good Menahga Finn, Ernst Huttah, is Dr. Wheaton's prized muscle therapist in Excelsior. Patients from the Falls, Bemidji area, Detroit

Lakes, Brainerd, flock to Menahga monthly for this three to six month treatment protocol to rehabilitate stretched, "wet noodle" (tensile overload of the joints) and are willing to pay out of pocket.

A few seasons ago, a Park Rapids basketball player avoided scheduled back surgery on a disc resulting from play. Football players and wrestlers from that area have also recovered and return to play unencumbered.

Nationwide high school, college, pro athletes get "welded" and sent back out with their team. After a full course of treatment, 3-6 sessions spaced monthly, athletes can expect to present to the coach next season with substantially repaired joints, often superior to pre-injury. Post-competition athletes, others injured from work or accident also benefit.

During the last Winter Olympics, Dr. Wheaton clarified on ESPN's "Outside the Lines" the legality and effectiveness of reconstructive injections after four American male skiers announced their use of Prolo, upsetting stuffed shirts on the Olympic committee who were not current in sports medicine.

If you are advised that this is "new, experimental or lacking in proof," that 'advisor' knows nothing about this sports medicine protocol which eliminates the cause of the pain, instead of masking the symptoms.

Thanks to Menahga, your athlete can have equal access to the best sports medicine taken for granted in the privileged southwestern suburbs, and thus perform at his/hers maximum capacity in this crucial developmental stage on his life.

Area Pioneer readers still express their gratitude for reporter Laurie Swenson's interview of Dr. Wheaton last April 14, 2006."

Arle Hagberg, Richard Leigh, M.D., (ret) Grand Forks

(Only auto insurance and workman's compensation automatically cover Prolo. With decent credit, check out www.CareCredit.com, for temporarily interest free, medical-only credit card. Dr. Wheaton is a participating doctor.)

What some of the Twins and The Utah Jazz have recently switched to:

A beverage derived from the Acai (assi – long "I") berry found in the flood plains of the Amazon Basin. One commercial brand is MonaVie, and comes in a 25 oz strong glass bottle. A separate formula is for pregnant women and children under ten years of age.

This beverage has been cleared for use by athletes by the president-elect of the NBA Physician's Association. The World Anti-Doping Agency has tested and proven MonaVie to be free of all banned substances. Athletes report a noticeable increase in speed, stamina and pain tolerance.

Single doses in gel form are available for convenient, safe storage in athletic bags. This 1-2 oz amount is consumed one hour prior to a game or workout and one hour following.

Recently a Minnesota college athlete suspected of a lung tumor was scheduled for surgery and for two weeks prior drank MonaVie daily. The day before surgery no trace of the suspicious growth could be medically observed and surgery was cancelled.

Other sources for this berry and other strong anti-oxidant formulas exist so explore your options and inquire of O.R.A.C. values, such as explained by Andrew Lessman and other reputable professionals.

ATTENTION ATHLETES:

Check out the pro hockey player Brian Pothier who credits special eye exercises for his return to the ice at www.covd.org.

This also benefitted a star wide receiver who excelled

in the 2009 Super Bowl – not on the winning team, however. Unfortunately, Ms. Hagberg cannot recall his name nor team, but in his interview he credited his grandfather who is an optometrist in Chicago.

His ability to catch 'just about any throw at any rate of speed from any angle' so impressed his team mates that THEY underwent this form of eye/hand exercise!

Appendix 6. JUST IN...

–Hope for Morgellons and Necrotizing Fasciitis

A good place to start, read the synopsis of George Noory's interview with Drs. Amelia Withington, Randy Wymore and Nurses James and Springstead on www.coasttocoastam.com for April 14, 2009.

These radio guests and patients describe the relief from intense itching, skin pain from non-toxic remedies, eg., Morgellons 'parasites' cannot tolerate hot/sour remedies such as heated vinegar, nor can they tolerate the patient's skin from being rubbed with plantain (plant) fibers. Certain Chelation doctors are involved as well.

Godspeed on your search,   www.thenmo.org/about.htm
For Necrotizing Fasciitis   www.nnff.org

Dr. Withington is board-certified by the American Board of Psychiatry and Neurology and has contracted Morgellons in the past.

–Summer, 2009, Ophthalmologist Edward Holland was featured on TBN's Doctor to Doctor, explaining his success with swabbing a cornea patient's mouth for stem cells, growing these in the lab, then transplanting them into the patients eye with complete success.

www.cincinnatieye.com

–Summer, 2009, U of MN Veterinary Surgeon Liz Pluhar successfully reversed 12 of 12 glioma brain tumors in canines using surgery and an auto-vaccine from each patient. See Poster Dog "Batman"

www.braintumorlab.com

...and finally,
Suzanne Sommers 'spills the beans' on Larry King Live

—with her latest publication, KNOCKOUT, interviews with leading alternative cancer specialists in the United States! She was allowed to speak out regarding her own full-body misdiagnosis of cancer in this Fall, 2009 special. On the same program:

CNN permitted interviews with Houston doctor Stanislaw Burzynski www.cancermed.com and Park Avenue, New York's Nick Gonzales, successful in pancreatic cancer www.dr-gonzales.com

Watch the following rising medical stars for their discoveries and listen for them on late night radio:

—Dr. Apsley's future e-books
www.drapsley.com.

His www.coasttocoast.com interview, February 2010, in which he describes Dr. Simoncini's use of sodium bicarbonate, baking soda, to destroy malignant tissue. Colleagues of Dr. Starr will also re-appear:

Dr. Mark Starr, March 9, 2010 interview with host George Noorie explains the emerging, more effective means to diagnose and treat Hypothyroid Type 2. For his book, medical practice www.21centurymed.com.

Dr. Jerry Tennant,
"Healing is voltage" medical expert
www.tennantinstitute.com.

Still want more? Go and
www.askwaltstoll.com!

YOUR NOTES:

Made in the USA
Middletown, DE
05 September 2021